Advanced Praise for *The Virtual Breastfeeding Culture*

In this digital age, mother-to-mother breastfeeding support has undergone a radical transformation. To understand this paradigm shift, and its impact on women and breastfeeding supporters, look no further than Lara Audelo's must-have resource, *The Virtual Breastfeeding Culture*. In it Audelo describes how social media connects soul mates struggling with a vast array of breastfeeding challenges: exclusive pumping, food sensitivities, tongue tie, low milk production, mood disorders, and more. She explains the deep emotional bonds mothers form and how they can often offset a lack of support in their "real" life, as well as insights into how breastfeeding supporters can most effectively tap into this powerful network.

--Nancy Mohrbacher, IBCLC, FILCA
Co-author, *Breastfeeding Made Simple: Seven Natural Laws for Nursing Mothers*

The Virtual Breastfeeding Culture
Seeking Mother-to-Mother Support in the Digital Age

Lara Audelo, CLEC

Praeclarus Press, LLC

www.PraeclarusPress.com

Praeclarus Press, LLC
2504 Sweetgum Lane
Amarillo, Texas 79124 USA
806-367-9950
www.PraeclarusPress.com

DISCLAIMER

The information contained in this publication is advisory only and is not intended to replace sound clinical judgment or individualized patient care. The author disclaims all warranties, whether expressed or implied, including any warranty as the quality, accuracy, safety, or suitability of this information for any particular purpose.

ISBN: 978-1-939807-02-1

ISBN (e-book): 978-1-939807-03-8

Cover Design: Ken Tackett
Developmental Editing: Kathleen Kendall-Tackett
Copy Editing: Diana Cassar-Uhl
Layout & Design: Todd Rollison
Operations: Scott Sherwood

For many women, their virtual friends become more important than their local face-friends who are ignorant or disapproving. For them, the Internet is priceless.

-Kathy Dettwyler

This book is dedicated to the sisterhood, which is you and me, and every mother we meet who needs our help. Our collective experiences and knowledge can serve to guide and support her, and help her arrive in the confident place she deserves to be.

Table of Contents

Foreword   9

Acknowledgements   12

Introduction   13

Chapter 1
The Pioneers of Online Breastfeeding
Support   21

Chapter 2
Caught by the Booby Traps®   25

Chapter 3
Pumping and Working   39

Chapter 4
A Mother's Loss: Breastfeeding After
Losing a Child   51

Chapter 5
Breastfeeding Preemies in the NICU   61

Chapter 6
Food Sensitivities   75

Chapter 7
Exclusive Pumpers   83

Chapter 8
Milk Donors   97

Chapter 9
Too Little, Too Much: IGT and BFAR   107

Chapter 10
All Tied Up: Tongue Tie and Lip Tie   125

Chapter 11
Breastfeeding with Depression and Mood
Disorders   139

Chapter 12
The Unexpected While Pregnant   153

Chapter 13
How the Lactation Professional Connects:
Why Social Media is Necessary for
Today's IBCLCs   171

Resources   187

References   201

Foreword

As two mothers who frequently curse the smart phones in our children's (and our own!) hands, and who bemoan the negative impact of technology on manners and relationship skills, it might seem contradictory that we would write a foreword for a book extolling online breastfeeding support. After all, we still mourn the days before the industrial revolution, when most extended families lived close together, and breastfeeding wisdom was passed down, in person, from mother to mother, or tribal healer to patient. There's still no "app" for a hug, or crying on another mother's shoulder.

There's also the grim reality that businesses have become savvier on leveraging the Internet to reach and influence expecting and new mothers far faster than health professionals have been able to keep pace. Whereas before we only had to contend with misleading advice and ads in magazines and formula freebies in hospitals, we're horrified that now innocent mothers can type "breastfeeding" into a search engine and be inundated with formula freebies and offers, their every move tracked by "cookies." The predatory and aggressive marketing practices that shattered the mother-to-daughter circle of breastfeeding support have infiltrated the Internet too. Formula-company-sponsored ads promising "expert feeding help" are embedded deeply into the breastfeeding guides of some popular websites, reaching millions of readers per month.

Fortunately, the Internet cuts both ways, and savvy mothers have learned to leverage it to help level the playing field. Necessity is the mother of invention (and mothers are pretty darn inventive), so they have found or created their own support system to overcome the lack of intergenerational woman-to-woman support and intra-peer network that once existed to help them learn the ropes of breastfeeding. With breastfeeding having taken a backseat to bottle-feeding in the last 70+ years, today's mothers need untraditional ways to find a tribe of like-minded women to help them navigate the myriad cultural, legal, and institutional barriers—the Booby Traps®—that continuously threaten to undermine them. Even for new mothers who are lucky enough to have supportive family members or communities nearby, the Internet offers more than information: Internet support groups offer anonymity, patience, and acceptance. Twitter friends understand if you don't respond right away, there is likely to be a Facebook page for every issue you about which you may be embarrassed to tell anyone you really know in person, and you can always exit a thread or discussion that doesn't meet your needs.

Being a public forum, social media tends to accelerate a group conscience shift toward helpful support. A negative or judgmental comment is likely to bring out the tigress in a protective Twitter or Facebook friend, with the unexpected outcome that a whole slew of users, followers or commenters get educated about breastfeeding support ethics in a flash.

That's not to say there aren't pitfalls. We've seen an atrocious lack of manners and restraint in some comment strings on controversial stories, and the occasional advocacy conversation derailed by personal attacks. But for the most part, support networks are filled with love and understanding, and today's mothers know how to find the Facebook page or discussion forum where they feel most comfortable. Finding a safe haven is key to growth and stretching beyond one's comfort zone in adopting healthy new behaviors.

The Internet has also given rise to a new form of activism; those mothers passionate about overcoming their own breastfeeding hurdles are now creating campaigns to help other mothers through sites like Change.org or Care2.com. Organizations like Best for Babes, MomsRising, and the United States Breastfeeding Committee are leveraging the Internet community to engage more mothers and advocates, influence the media, and effect policy change.

But breastfeeding support, and social change still starts one mother at a time, and in this wonderful book, Lara Audelo brings together powerful stories of how social media and the Internet have helped individual mothers overcome barriers and find resources to succeed. Lara's deep passion for nurturing, breastfeeding, and parenting, and her insistence on academic rigor and evidence-based practice makes her a powerful advocate. Her vast experience of helping mothers online, and cheering them on, makes her an authority on using social media for social good. Her personality comes alive in social media. Her wicked sense of humor and wizardry with e-cards pepper her Facebook posts and Tweets, bringing much-needed laughter where there were tears, and provoking discussion and sowing the seeds for action. It's hard to find someone in the breastfeeding world who has not been touched by Lara's wit, wisdom, and warmth, whether personally, in a advocacy conversation, or through her "Peace. Love. Breastfeeding." T-shirts. We are deeply grateful that all of her talents can reach a wider audience thanks to the 'Net!

Mothers who read this book will find validation in their experiences, and a wider lens through which they will be better able to support their friends. Healthcare professionals will find proof that we need to meet mothers where they are at—both physically and emotionally—especially since there are fewer enrollees in traditional birth classes and a burgeoning of chat groups online. The Internet is a zone of connectivity governed by somewhat different terms of engagement, and this book will open the doors to understanding the new playing field. Anyone who works with expecting or new mothers will find encouragement, resources, and helpful guidelines for how to support new mothers online. *The Virtual Breastfeeding Culture* is a clarion call to change the way we support expecting and new mothers, and is a valuable addition to the breastfeeding-support library!

Danielle Rigg, JD, CLC and Bettina Forbes, CLC
Best for Babes Foundation

Acknowledgements

My deepest gratitude to my amazingly supportive friends and family; my sister for being there for me as a best friend and mothering role model, and my Aunt Trisha, who tells me every time I share a big dream with her, "Sweetie you can do anything you put your mind to!" I could not have come this far without the love, encouragement, and help of my husband and children. I'll always be eternally grateful to my two boys, who taught me just how special breastfeeding could be. Without the experience loving them through breastfeeding and nursing them thousands of times over the last six years, I never would have found the work that makes me so passionate.

I am so very fortunate to work with amazing people who have provided me with incredible opportunities. They serve as both friends and mentors, and I am forever grateful for every morsel of knowledge they share with me. I hope to never stop learning from their experience and to always have access to their wisdom.

Amber McCann, Robin Kaplan, and Fleur Bickford, thank you for saying yes without hesitation when I asked for your help in reaching professionals with the final chapter of this book. Your insight on this subject is beyond valuable and will benefit so many mothers and professionals. Also an incredibly deep, heart-felt thank you to Kathleen Kendall-Tackett, who said yes when I pitched her this book idea, and offered me nothing but support and guidance as I navigated the uncharted waters of this project.

Lastly, for all the mothers who took the time to tell us their stories, and mustered the courage to relive and share such intimate details of their experiences, I will always be grateful for your trusting me with these pieces of yourselves.

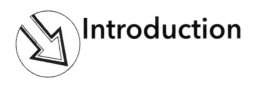 # Introduction

My Story: Finding Help and Making Friends Online

I can't recall ever seeing women breastfeed their babies when I was growing up. To be honest, there weren't many babies around me at all when I was a child. I was the youngest in my family, and my sister is four and a half years older. Neither one of us was ever into playing with dolls, so we didn't walk around and mimic breastfeeding as you will see some little girls do with their babies. I know my grandmother breastfed my mother and my uncle, my mom breastfed my sister and me for a short time, but both of us were pioneers when it came to our own breastfeeding relationships with our children, specifically with regard to the duration that we chose to breastfeed our children. I always knew that if I had children I wanted to breastfeed, but I never really gave much thought to all it would entail before I was pregnant.

Once I learned I was pregnant with my older son in May 2006, I began to research everything from natural childbirth to breastfeeding. I enjoy digging for information, and I rarely make a decision without weighing the options after examining a good bit of research. For me, birth and breastfeeding were no different. I must give credit to my sister though because she was really the one who brought breastfeeding out of "captivity" for me as she breastfed my nieces anytime, anywhere. Both of them weaned well into their preschool years. Without her as an example, I am fairly certain I would not have made it to 70 months and counting in my breastfeeding career.

Based on what I had read, I decided it was in my best interest to write a birth plan, take childbirth classes, and hire a doula to assist me in giving birth. Looking back, I realize that my birth choices were almost completely motivated by my desire to successfully breastfeed. My sister and I talked about childbirth. She discussed her drug-free births with me at length and she said, "You will only have a couple chances to ever feel the sensation of pushing your baby into the world, and it really is something you shouldn't miss." That sentiment resonated with me, and after two unmedicated births, I am so thankful she shared it with me.

When it was time for my son to make his arrival, everything went as planned: no epidural, short pushing stage, and only a first degree tear. I really was lucky for a woman having her first baby in a hospital that had a 98% epidural rate, and was not afraid of interventions. But we did have an unforeseen hiccough as soon as my son was born: he was taken to the Neonatal Intensive Care Unit (NICU) for two days because he had difficulty breathing immediately after birth, and was diagnosed with a pneumothorax. Thankfully, he recovered quickly and we both went home at the 48-hour mark. His NICU stay was something for which I had not planned, and it meant that I had to deal with a few unsupportive members of the hospital staff. It also meant that I had to really stand my ground when it came to the fact that because I was pumping colostrum for him, he did not need to be supplemented with formula. He was about 27 hours old when I first put him to my breast, and he took to it like a champ.

During this time, I did have something to be very grateful for in this instance: my sister had driven from her home, about two hours away, to sit with me in the NICU and to help me breastfeed him for the first time. I received help from a couple of the nurses, but because it was the weekend, there was not a lactation consultant on duty, and it was not a Baby-Friendly Hospital; there was plenty of free formula being used and given out. The point is, I only had my sister. My first birth was before everyone had smartphones and could access the Internet from their pockets. It was before Facebook had millions of users and thousands of breastfeeding-support pages. It was before Twitter was accessible from anything other than a computer. If not for the support of my sister, with her real-life breastfeeding experience, breastfeeding would not have been so easy. My sister not only gave me technical breastfeeding advice, her presence gave me confidence and helped me feel secure, which were priceless to me as a new mother learning to breastfeed.

Shortly after my son was born, our little family of three re-located from the East Coast to the West Coast, and I found myself in a new place with no friends, a husband who was gone on deployment, a four month-old baby, and still many, many questions as a new mother. When my son was about six months old, I turned to the Internet for breastfeeding support. Looking back, it was a watershed moment for me. I had no idea that so much of my time would include helping breastfeeding mothers through the Internet, and using technology to help mothers feel confident, the way my sister helped me as I sat in the NICU with my new baby. But that is exactly what happened. I turned to the La Leche League International mother-to-mother forums to ask a question and quickly got an answer from a handful of moms. I then asked another question, and before I knew it, I was asking for advice and offering advice to other breastfeeding mothers with questions. Then something unexpected happened; I was making friends in a way that I never had before—online.

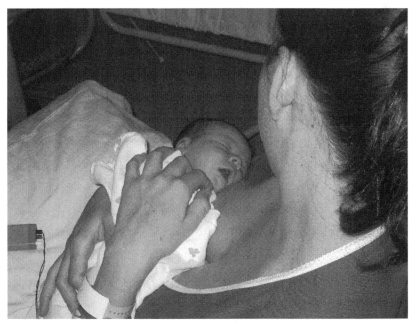

My older son's first "milk coma" after breastfeeding successfully in the NICU at 27 hours old. —*Photo credit: Lara Audelo*

My Second Birth

My second son was born in the summer of 2009, and my early breastfeeding experience with him was very different. His birth was wonderful as well; he was placed directly on my chest and latched on and began breastfeeding within about ten minutes after birth. Having had two very different experiences made it possible for me to relate to more mothers, and I quickly realized that breastfeeding counseling and education was a professional avenue I wanted to pursue. I suppose the fact that it all happened online was serendipitous; because I had two young children and a husband who was deployed often, working outside of the home was not an option for our family. I did what I knew best; I hooked up to the Internet and began connecting with other breastfeeding mothers, to offer support, encouragement and advice. Mother-to-mother support is something I firmly believe you really can never have enough of. I have never heard a mother say, "You know I have had way too many people offer to help me breastfeed successfully. Thanks, but no thanks!" Even veteran moms have questions.

The Advantages of Online Support

The Internet offers support in a unique way: you can take what you want and leave the rest. You can walk away at any time, or you can find mothers online at 2 a.m. when you are in need of support and encouragement for another late-night feeding that has left you feeling ragged. It's a global community, after all, and your 2 a.m. is someone else's 10 a.m. You might find like-minded women who share many of the same values, who live in a different town, state, or country–but your similarities are enough that you form friendships and keep coming back for more support.

If you don't have access to local support groups at hospitals, or there are no breastfeeding mothers who meet regularly in your area, then you don't have to be alone; you can find your tribe online. The collective group of online mothers offering nursing support is very giving. Someone will hop in on a moment's notice to help. Access is instant, and in our increasingly technologically driven world, this is appealing to many mothers. Sometimes the support becomes real and tangible: a card for Christmas, a birthday present, a sympathy gift for a lost relative, etc. Either way, the friendships are real and the support is invaluable. Online support helped me to continue breastfeeding, and on some days my online support group saved my sanity!

As we will see in the next chapter, The Pioneers of Online Breast-feeding Support, women came to the Internet first to support one another. That is pretty impressive: we learned and mastered new technology, found a way to use it for our benefit and growth, and established an online presence that has grown exponentially. Once organizations and industry saw where we were, they followed us into cyberspace. Let it be known that women came to the Internet first and we were not drawn here by others wanting to support us. Today, finding breastfeeding on the Web is a no-brainer. Anyone who wants to connect with mothers knows this is where we can be found. Even the U. S. Surgeon General, Dr. Regina Benjamin, pointed out in her 2011 *Call to Action to Support Breastfeeding* that, "the increasing use of electronic communication channels opens up new possibilities for supporting breastfeeding" (cited in McCann & McCulloch, 2012, p. 450)

Mothers have been using the Internet to help one another since the 1990s, but those born after 1982, which we refer to as the Millennial Generation, grew up alongside the Internet, and they use technology in almost every aspect of their lives. Time spent online increases after our babies are born by as much as 44% (McCann & McCulloch, 2012). A recent study, Feeding on the Web: Online Social Support in the Breastfeeding Context, by Jennifer Gray, examines how and why women are plugging into the virtual world for breastfeeding support.

> More and more women are turning to the Web for health-related support, making it a fruitful option to study breastfeeding communication ... An interesting arena to study breastfeeding support communication is the Internet as it offers a record of such support requested and received, and is a place more and more women are seeking breastfeeding support and information (Gray, 2013).

One of the advantages of Internet support is that there is probably more information available than one could ever obtain in a lifetime, especially when you consider that the body of resources is constantly growing. With every breastfeeding-related article published, blog post shared, question answered on a Facebook Timeline, or tweet sent through the "Twitterverse," this information is stored and can be accessed at will when needed by mothers. The best part is that once you connect with mothers online, they will show you exactly where to go to get what you need. Then that mother will share it, and so on and so on. In less than two decades, women have built an amazing virtual infrastructure of support with the hope that no mother in need of help will fall through the cracks.

One aspect of virtual support, which every story in this book shares, is that mothers came to the Internet for answers, and they often stayed because of friends. Friendships began online with the first groups of women who communicated through email and LISTSERVs, and they became more real with the passage of time as technology now allows women to share not only stories, but pictures and videos of themselves and their families, thus enhancing the "real-life" aspect of virtual friendships. It should come as no surprise that women in the early days of motherhood spend more time online than ever before.

> They may participate in hyperpersonal communication online, building relationships and finding support that they could not receive face to face, particularly those who are isolated in the early period after a birth, feeding an infant at home every two to three hours (Gray, 2013).

Ask any new mother who is at home with a week-old baby how different her life is now, and she probably wouldn't even be able to articulate the incredible change. It is an awkward time. We need support and help more than ever, but we are often alone and afraid because we have no idea what we are doing.

Here are our stories. We all define success in our own way, and we all reached out and received valuable support through the Internet, whether that was by using social media, like Facebook and Twitter, or by reading blogs about breastfeeding written by both lactation professionals and breastfeeding mothers, using forums, or email LISTSERVs. No mother should ever feel alone, or feel like she doesn't have anyone to talk to and ask questions, and technology has given us a way to end the isolation and increase support: anywhere, anytime.

Chapter 1

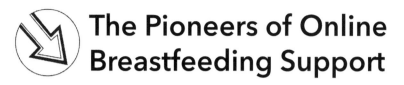 The Pioneers of Online
Breastfeeding Support

In the early-to-mid 1990s, the world became a lot smaller, so to speak, as the masses discovered the Internet. It was the beginning of being able to sit on your couch and "surf the Web!" I will never forget my first Internet experience. It was 1995. I was a sophomore in college and taking an anthropology class. The professor wanted to show us something about cave paintings in Lascaux, France. He went to the computer, typed a URL into the browser bar, and off we went to France! I was amazed.

At the same time as I was using the Internet in college, my older sister, Lisa, was using it to gain the breastfeeding support she wasn't finding in person. My oldest niece was born in 1995, and at four months old had to have cranial surgery. Lisa turned online for support and found a group of mothers she could relate to, who turned into her friends. At the time, she was rather new to where she was living, and needed connections. She was well-researched about breastfeeding and babies from reading books, but books can't carry on conversations and empathize with the challenges of being a new mother. The Internet provided her breastfeeding and mothering support. Long before the age of social media, or even forums, Lisa was simply connected through emails. Every day mothers would write each other with questions, issues, and concerns. These questions were not always about breastfeeding, but that is what brought them together in the first place.

I've spoken with other mothers who used the Internet in its early days, and they said the same thing: their online connections gave them a strong sense of belonging when they had no "real life" support. Parent-L, an international group formed a LISTSERV for breastfeeding and Attachment Parenting, and drew many mothers. Some were open about their involvement, while others kept their online lives more private. Today, it's probably hard to imagine not sharing an online presence—especially when we share everything from pictures of our dinner to our children's first birthday parties, but in the early days of Internet usage, some women chose to keep their involvement in online support groups private because others who weren't making valuable Internet connections just couldn't understand these virtual friendships. Interestingly, all of the mothers I asked who relied on the Internet credit these early online resources as almost life-saving, and with creating and helping them maintain lifelong friendships. Marisa Steffers, an original Parent-L member said of her friends:

> ... what we have is magical, really ... we've had births, and deaths, and breast-cancer diagnoses, 9/11. I've met, in real life I think seven women from the list, and we share books, and joys, and sorrows ... the women at Parent-L are smart, thoughtful, kind ...

This aspect of virtual help hasn't changed, as you will see. Even though social media has made communication more sophisticated, it hasn't changed the value women give to their online networks.

Kathy Dettwyler, one of the most respected, well-known lactation experts working in the field today, was part of this early group of mothers on Parent-L. She continued to support mothers online in the 1990s, even though she was no longer nursing.

> Remember, by the time the Internet came along, I had nursed three kids and spent my career doing research on breastfeeding, including speaking at conferences, and writing articles and books. I was the one providing support. I set up a website, with lots of articles and links (Kathy Dettwyler, personal communication, January 6, 2013)

Kathy's website is still one of the most popular and well-visited sites today (www.kathydettwyler.org).

Almost two decades ago, establishing a website, or even starting a LISTSERV was not something that just anyone could do. Hanna Graeffe, a Parent-L member from Finland, recognized by one of the biggest baby magazines in her country as an online pioneer of breast-feeding support, noted: "You had to know someone from a university" to establish a LISTSERV. Almost 20 years later, when you look at the legacy of LISTSERVs with regard to breastfeeding support, we see more than long-lasting friendships. Groups of women, who emerged as key players fueled by their passion, used the Internet to give rise to global breastfeeding activism we know and embrace today. Hanna shared that in Finland:

> The National Breastfeeding Association started form-ing and growing from that list, and now the asso-ciation has several employees, and a position as the breastfeeding expert in this country; and there are plenty of support groups, both real-life and online available, and a national phone line you can call for breastfeeding support. All this came from the breastfeeding email list! (Hanna Graeffe, personal communication, January 6, 2013)

It's difficult to measure the value of these early online methods of breastfeeding support. Looking back, Kathy Dettwyler notes:

> The Internet has, of course, revolutionized informa-tion access and sharing. Now there are lots of places for people to get help and info and support. Of course, at the same time, this means that conflicting information is out there on almost any topic related to breastfeeding, and a lot of misinformation is also out there. So it's been a mixed blessing (Personal communication, January 6, 2013).

In the last decade the emergence of widely used social media platforms has forever changed how we live in our world: everything is instant and we are always connected. We are never far away from anyone, even if they are literally half a world away. As a breastfeeding mother, the ability to get the answers we need in real time can make all the difference in helping you achieve your breastfeeding goals.

Chapter 2

Caught by the Booby Traps®

When I put out the call for stories of online breastfeeding support to be submitted for this book, I received hundreds of responses from mothers willing to share their experiences, each one with a unique story. The book easily became organized based on the common elements the mothers' stories shared. Many women struggled from the very beginning, lacking support around them to help them breastfeed successfully. Sometimes they were able to make it work in spite of these hurdles. Other times, they weren't capable of meeting their breastfeeding goals.

Some mothers face everyday breastfeeding struggles—a hospital that sends her away with free formula instead of lactation support, an employer who doesn't allow for pumping breaks while at work, family members who don't understand why they can't just feed the new baby a bottle. These challenges, either alone or combined, can doom breastfeeding relationships, but these are obstacles that can be prevented or remedied with education and support. We can inform the staff at the hospital about the dangers of unnecessary formula supplementation. We can push for better legislation to support breastfeeding mothers in the workplace. And we can educate families about how even one ill-timed bottle of formula to make a mother-in-law happy can lead to breastfeeding cessation. The Best for Babes Foundation® calls these preventable hindrances that mother/baby dyads face Booby Traps®. Among breastfeeding circles and groups, the phrase "Booby Traps" has become part of the vernacular, and these hurdles come in all shapes and sizes, such as in the examples above. Best for Babes' co-founders Bettina Forbes and Danielle Rigg classify Booby Traps as either cultural or institutional. It's not an overstatement to say that in the United States, various combinations of the two lie in the path of every woman who breastfeeds. We see and hear these stories over and over again. Mothers say, "I just couldn't produce enough milk," or "My employer wouldn't give me adequate time and space to pump." We know that some moms don't actually produce enough milk; but the majority can, and employers can be educated about laws protecting breastfeeding mothers. Education can address many of these issues. We should not blame mothers for being Booby Trapped. Blaming mothers fosters maternal guilt, which is counterproductive, and is unfair to women. Moreover, blame will never change the system, but education can.

Reading this, you may not know how you were Booby Trapped, but perhaps reading these stories will help you figure it out. Every mother is at risk for being caught by at least one. However, if we share our experiences, support one another, and work to educate not only parents, but everyone who is involved in making breastfeeding work (employers, family, healthcare providers), we can hopefully eliminate the Booby Traps once and for all.

Maya's Story

I had not really been exposed to breastfeeding prior to graduate school. My mother nursed my younger siblings and me, but I don't have memory of her doing so, nor can I recall seeing other women breastfeed. However, during the first quarter of my Master of Public Health program, I was assigned the topic of researching breastfeeding-rate disparities. It opened my mind to some of the misinformation about breastfeeding, as well as cultural beliefs surrounding the decision on how to feed your baby. Even then, I knew I still had a lot to learn! When I became pregnant later that year I decided, as a result of that project, that I would breastfeed my child for six months. Looking back, I knew very little, only that I did not want my child to have formula or a pacifier in the hospital.

My son's birth didn't go as I'd hoped. At 37 weeks, I was told that I needed a planned c-section under general anesthesia due to a problem with my spine, and it was scheduled for 39 weeks. After he was delivered, I woke up on the telemetry unit, where I learned that I'd had a complication during the surgery. My son, Miles, was in the newborn nursery and he'd been given formula for low blood sugar and low body temperature. I was upset that he'd had formula against our wishes, but my husband had been assured that it was necessary. I begged a nurse—to the point of sobbing—for her to bring my baby boy to me so I could nurse him. She did a couple of times that night, but he was apparently blocked from seeing me after that until the next afternoon, when I was moved to the newborn floor. I was extremely distressed, and looking back, I now see this was our first Booby Trap!

Luckily, Miles latched easily and nursed well, though I felt awkward and embarrassed breastfeeding, especially as we had a slew of visitors coming in and out. The only cover I had was the big blanket on the bed, and there are photos of me trying to nurse with both Miles and me hidden by the blanket over my head. That second evening, a nurse informed me that I was not supposed to be breastfeeding while on the medication I was taking. She brought me a pump and taught me how to pump my milk while I gave Miles formula. Once this mistake was finally cleared up, I was allowed to nurse again. But then the hospital's pediatrician told me Miles had lost too much weight and I should supplement. Here I was, Booby Trapped again! I remembered a friend telling me that it's normal for a newborn to lose up to 10% of his body weight after birth, so I told the pediatrician this and refused to go back to the formula.

We had a few other pitfalls after that, but nothing daunting. Three weeks after Miles's birth, we picked up and moved across the country. It was at this point, as a new mom living far from home with no friends, that I turned to social media. At first, I wasn't asking breastfeeding questions, just developing relationships. I met some "lactivists," but stayed away from most of their breastfeeding talk. They might feel comfortable nursing in public, but not me! No, I pumped milk and brought it with me when I went out. And if I couldn't do that then I had a cover. And nursing on demand? That sounded awful! No, I was just fine thank you very much!

When Miles was seven months old, my cardiologist and I decided to change my heart medication, and I was instructed that to do so I needed to wean Miles. I received little direction on how to wean. The two-week process was physically and emotionally painful, from the hormone changes, engorgement, comments I got online questioning my decision, and the lack of being ready to end the nursing relationship on both Miles's and my parts. I realized that breastfeeding was a whole lot more important to me than I'd ever thought it would be.

I started reading more of the articles that those breastfeeding advocates tweeted, and as I did so, I realized I agreed with what they were saying. Six months later, I became pregnant and convinced my husband, at the suggestion of my online friends, that I needed to hire a doula for the birth of our second son. Miles's birth had been traumatic for me, and I decided I wanted a VBAC and the immediate breastfeeding experience that others had. I can honestly say I would never have considered a VBAC if it hadn't been for a few women online who opened my mind and allayed my fears with facts.

I felt so much more prepared and at peace that second time around. Through Twitter, Facebook, and articles online, I learned what questions to ask my OBGYN in order to feel like an equal part of the decision-making team. When complications arose, I knew I had my Twitter friends to support me. In the end, I needed to have a c-section. Unlike with Miles's birth though, I felt at peace that this c-section was necessary for my son's well being. My husband was able to watch Julian being born, go with him to the nursery, and with help from my doula, I was breastfeeding Julian about a half hour after his birth. It was beautiful!

Other than a short visit from an IBCLC, I did not get any breastfeeding support during the five days I spent in the hospital. My husband actually had to request a different nurse at one point because the one I had was giving me a hard time about breastfeeding. I asked my online friends, both directly and via Twitter using the #bfcafe hashtag, many questions while I was in the hospital. My husband and I also made the decision to have Julian room-in with us instead of going to the nursery, and not to not allow any visitors, save Miles and my grandmother, in order to give me time to feel comfortable breastfeeding. Because of the Booby Traps I experienced with Miles, I was prepared to dodge them all when I had Julian!

After I got home, Julian continued to have trouble latching, most likely due to his high-arch palate. A Twitter friend found an IBCLC for me near where I lived, and she was invaluable! She gave me a small SNS to supplement Julian with using my pumped milk, and showed me tricks to strengthen his latch. It was a difficult five weeks, but eventually he was nursing like a champ! I felt so much more confident nursing Julian too. Soon after he was born I was nursing in restaurants, at church, the doctor's office—without a cover!

Thanks to Social Media support, I've learned the best way to treat thrush (which Julian and I have gotten too many times to count), what baby-led weaning is, and how to gently night wean. In turn, I've since been able to provide support and information to friends and women online, via email, Facebook, and Twitter. I love #bfcafe and the website KellyMom (www.kellymom.com) in particular. I had a goal of exclusively breastfeeding Julian for one year. As I write this, we've been breastfeeding for 25 months, something I never thought I'd want to do before I became connected to the online breastfeeding community.

If you're considering looking for breastfeeding information or support online, it's a great choice! I know that the information I've received, and the friends I've made have influenced multiple aspects of my parenting. Make sure that you're getting reliable information, though. Look for sources that cite facts—not opinions. Surround yourself with people who listen and offer evidence-based advice, and not people who are going to be judgmental. I believe that most any feeding choice is viable, but that it should be an informed choice, and you should feel comfortable.

Jaimie's Story

My story really begins with my first daughter, whom I was not able to breastfeed. I had a relatively normal pregnancy, except for the fact that I was diagnosed with gestational diabetes, which really affected my birth experience. Because of the gestational diabetes, I was advised that I needed to be induced at 40 weeks. My body and baby weren't ready, and the induction led to a 17-hour-long cascade of interventions, ending in a c-section. We believe all of her thrashing around during the induction caused her to wrap the cord around her neck three times, and she ended up with a pneumothorax (air bubble trapped outside of her lung). Babies with this condition are routinely observed in the NICU. She ended up spending two days there, and wasn't allowed to eat for the first 24 hours. I began a regular pumping schedule to help my milk come in, and the NICU stored it for us. When they declared she could finally eat, I couldn't get down there right away, and there wasn't time to thaw my frozen milk, so her first meal was a bottle of formula. We tried numerous times to get her to latch before we left the NICU, but without success. One nurse was able to "pop her on" once–and only once—so Mikki nursed from me for about ten minutes. That's the only time she ever did.

I tried to work with the one lactation consultant at the hospital, but they were understaffed and she only had about ten minutes to spend with me. To make our breastfeeding even more difficult, Mikki had jaundice and had to stay an extra day after I was released. From the first bottle of formula to the absence of lactation support, we fell victim to the snowball effect of Booby Traps. Due to difficulty healing and exhaustion, I was only able to pump for a total of three weeks, so my supply dwindled and she was fed formula permanently.

During my pregnancy with Mikki, I joined an online "due date" club, where I met a number of ladies, a couple of them with whom I am still very close. One of them, Amy, had a difficult pregnancy, but wanted to breastfeed. After two days she was ready to give up–it hurt too much, etc. Thankfully, she received valuable lactation support, and went on breastfeed for more than two years! She even became a breastfeeding advocate and Certified Lactation Counselor because of her positive experience. Even though I was far from being pregnant again, Amy proved to be an inspiration and a valuable resource to me in the future.

When I did become pregnant the second time I was determined to make it work. During my first pregnancy, I always figured, "Hey, it's natural. It should be easy to do." My mother breastfed my brother and me when we were babies, and had sought help from La Leche League. Today, technology made finding support much easier. By this time, my due-date club had moved to Facebook, along with a lot of my other friends. I discovered pages like The Leaky Boob (www.facebook.com/TheLeakyBoob), which offered all kinds of mother-

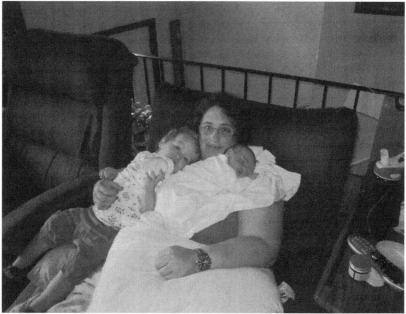

Jaimie snuggling with her daughter, proud that she beat the Booby Traps® on her second try! — *Photo credit: Jaimie Leader-Goodale*

to-mother advice, and I started talking to Amy about breastfeeding preparation. I was able to use the web to search for an IBCLC this time. The first time I didn't even know what an IBCLC was! I was able to interview them over the phone, and I was prepared with my own consultant in case the hospital was overwhelmed again. She and I stayed in contact via email and Facebook throughout my pregnancy, and she came to the hospital two hours after I gave birth to be there, and support me, and make sure I was in good shape. She also brought me a rental pump so I could have it when I was ready to start pumping, and was always there for me whenever I had questions. Facebook groups, online friends, and Internet resources all pooled together and afforded me the opportunity to breastfeed my youngest daughter for 17 months.

Were there other factors contributing to my success besides the Internet? Of course. For one thing this birth was a scheduled c-section, as I had gestational diabetes again, and we didn't want to risk the possible health issues of another failed induction. There wasn't the much harder healing I had experienced after my induction, and I was able to heal and function much more quickly. Also, I was determined to fix what went wrong the last time.

The availability of resources through social media, the Internet, and email made success a much-more-likely possibility. The friends I've made through this process are still with me, and my experiences are what inspired me to start a business supporting breastfeeding mothers. I hope that stories like mine will help new mothers and mothers-to-be realize that help is out there, and you aren't failing if you need to seek help. We're out here, countless mothers who have been through similar experiences, survived the Booby Traps, and who will help and guide others along the way.

Rachel's Story

The most exposure I had to breastfeeding before becoming a mother was during our CenteringPregnancy class. At the time, my husband and I were living in Manhattan, KS, as my husband is Active Duty Army and was stationed at Ft. Riley. We received our prenatal care through Irwin Army Community Hospital (IACH). CenteringPregnancy was a wonderful support and informational group. IACH's lactation consultant came during the breastfeeding session, and that was pretty much the very first time I considered the question of whether we were going to breastfeed. An extended-family breast-cancer situation, coupled with my husband and I going vegan during month six of my pregnancy, set my mind completely to breastfeed no matter what it took from me to do so.

I was working full-time during my pregnancy and started my maternity leave on Week 38. My job consisted of 40 hours on my feet bustling around a large retail store, so the extra time off was necessary for my sanity and energy at that point. My pregnancy was uneventful and healthy.

The day before we hit Week 41, we had our non-stress test, which our son passed without a problem; however, the ultrasound showed an extremely low fluid level, so they admitted me immediately, and within two hours I was receiving Pitocin to induce labor. Fourteen hours later our son was born. It was a non-medicated, vaginal, relatively uneventful birth.

We did allow him to be wiped off and his APGAR taken in the same room. Within the hour, he was placed on my chest, and my nurse began to assist us in our first breastfeeding session. I remember her being very hands-on, directing me, and manipulating him in an attempt to get him latched on. I'm not sure if he was sleepy, or if we would have been able to figure it out if we had relaxed or tried a Biological Nurturing approach, but what did end up happening was that the nurse declared I had flat nipples and promptly placed a nipple shield on me.

Everything seemed to be going okay. Unfortunately, the hospital lactation consultant was out of town that weekend, so the extent of my breastfeeding support came from the random nurses that came in to check on me. They each offered advice, most of which worried and confused me. I was told to never let the baby use me as a pacifier and to use a pacifier instead. Then I was told to never deny the baby when he seemed to want to eat/drink, to "feed on demand," allowing him to get his sucking satisfaction on me. I was told to make sure I never ever fell asleep while nursing him; then a nurse showed me how to feed him side-lying. One nurse told me her friend's breasts became two different sizes and to make sure I fed him off of each side equally; then I was told to not worry about timing his feedings on each side too much. I was told nursing was a great, easy way to get baby to sleep; but I was not to let him sleep while nursing. At this point, I began my quest for breastfeeding support online.

The very first item I searched for was information about nipple shields, since one of the nurses commented that they were terrible things to use, and I needed to stop using them immediately. She did not provide any specifics as to how not to use it, though. The nurse who assisted at his birth and first nursing had proclaimed I had flat nipples, and it stuck in my head like a dire diagnosis. I couldn't fathom that with such an "ailment," I could not use the shield. I felt as if maybe my body wasn't made to feed my child, that maybe I was in that one to five percent of the population who truly cannot physiologically breastfeed. I can't recall what sites I ended up on at that time, but I do remember nursing my newborn and holding my iPod, frantically typing with one hand and reading all I could about what exactly I should be doing regarding feeding this baby, what was normal, what nipple shields were all about.

For the first month with our newborn, I spent the night feedings, and many day feedings, online reading up on "normal" newborn breastfeeding habits, quirks, routines, et cetera. I became very familiar with KellyMom, and I am nearly sure I have read every single article she's written, and most of all the links she provided as references. I spent some time on Ask Dr. Sears (www.AskDrSears.com), reading articles on breastfeeding, sleep development, and co-sleeping. I found Dr. McKenna's website (www.cosleeping.nd.edu/). He's in charge of the mother-infant sleep lab at Notre Dame and has a lot of great evidence-based information about breastfeeding and co-sleeping safety. I also found the Best for Babes Foundation, where I got a lot of information regarding nursing in public and pumping-at-work policy information.

I would mostly Google terms or questions, and read the results. A few times, La Leche League International's Mother-to-Mother online forums would come up in the results, and right before I went back to work, I decided to join their forums. They were instrumental to my breastfeeding success, I believe. I posted questions about pumping and returning to work, about "normal" breastfeeding baby behavior, and issues with our baby's doctor (a family practitioner). It was through the forums and their website that I connected with my local La Leche League group, first in Kansas and later in Ohio.

I turned to online support because it was the easiest way for me to get the answers I needed. The only family that was able to provide first-hand experience and support was my cousin's wife; no other close family had breastfeeding experience. I was not keen on the lactation consultant at the hospital in Kansas, so the LLL leaders on the forums and locally were extremely helpful. My husband is incredibly supportive, and this upcoming year, while he's deployed and we live with family that is not always as supportive as I would like, will be interesting.

Online support has been the crux of our breastfeeding relationship. From the mothers online I learned how to dress to feed my baby in public without exposing my tummy or breast, how to nurse without using a cover, how to wean off the nipple shield, how to increase my pumping output when my supply regulated and I needed more milk, how to handle reverse-cycling, how to feed off the top breast while side-lying so there's no need to move my baby while sleeping, and how to nurse while wearing my baby in a variety of carriers. I still use the LLL forums and KellyMom's Facebook groups to receive support, and have questions and concerns addressed quickly.

To pregnant women, or new mothers, I would suggest that you treat searching for online breastfeeding support as you would if you were writing a research paper. Use professional, credentialed sites for the majority of your reading. Hearing and getting the opinions and experiences of other mothers can be helpful and reassuring, but it can also unwittingly be detrimental to your breastfeeding relationship. Remember that anecdotes are not necessarily reflective of the larger truth ("I did XYZ with my baby and everything's fine!" when research shows that XYZ is usually not helpful, so it's better to avoid XYZ if humanly possible).

No research, no amount of data can trump your intuition. If you turn off the noise of your mother, your in-laws, the baby books, the websites, the experts, and listen to your inner voice, she will lead you to what you need to know and do to raise (and feed) your baby the way your baby needs.

Toi's Story

Growing up, I don't ever recall seeing any mothers practice breastfeeding, or even anyone in my family doing it. I heard white people talk about it, but I never saw or heard anyone black talk about breastfeeding. Honestly, I can't even remember why I decided to breastfeed my first born, as I was young at the time. After being in labor for over 32 hours, I delivered a healthy 8lb 12oz baby girl. All I remember once she was born was that she was on my breast. I had no clue what was happening in my body, how milk was made, or my baby's important role in the process. Upon returning home from the hospital, I continued putting her to my breast while supplementing with formula. Understand, I had no clue about anything breastfeeding. I managed to breastfeed about six weeks, but with the lack of knowledge and support, I stopped. I didn't think she was getting full and she was very "colicky," or so people told me. On top of all this, I was returning to college and didn't know how she would be able to receive my milk while I was away.

Fast-forward five years; I was remarried and pregnant again. My loving husband and I decided that we would breastfeed, and thankfully my obstetrician was wonderful and supportive. He and his staff encouraged breastfeeding from our very first prenatal visit. They presented me with information on local breastfeeding resources, magazines, and online resources; I knew this time my experience would be different. I spent a great deal of time researching, and joked that I was probably overwhelming my hubby with all the information I was learning!

I joined some online "mommy" boards, like Babycenter.com and the La Leche League International (www.llli.org) Mother-to-Mother forums. I was so surprised at the information these other women had to share and stories they told. The moms were so helpful; we even emailed and exchanged phone numbers. These sites became my lifeline, and my husband often joked and laughed about me having more "online friends" than real-life ones. Websites, like KellyMom and Womenshealth.gov gave me what I called my "super power" to be successful with great reference information, as they explained so many things, including the most important thing: I had to make this my experience. Although there were shared stories, information, and facts, one theme was clear: that each mother-child relationship was different. I made sure I planned my goals accordingly, and didn't fear adjustments to that plan if they were needed. By the time I gave birth, I had a birthing plan, breastfeeding plan, return-to-work plan, and a well-informed supporting husband–and I gained all of this knowledge from my online resources. I knew what to expect, what to do, what not to do, and who to call for support or help.

After I gave birth, I felt more confident about breastfeeding because I knew what to expect: the first week, the growth spurts, the cluster feeds, etc. I was able to successfully breastfeed for about five months with no artificial milk, and then until he was 10 months using both, as I learned I was pregnant again. After breastfeeding successfully, I knew I could do it again with my next baby, and that I could call upon my resources as needed. That doesn't mean I didn't have issues, but I knew where to go to get help. In addition to all my online support, this time I can say extended family was more supportive. I think they finally understood that nothing they could say would change my mind about nursing my babies.

Breastfeeding was one of the greatest experiences of my life. Even after my last child self-weaned, I continued to educate myself and share this information with others. I offered assistance to moms in my church, work, and even on social media. I eventually became a breastfeeding peer counselor at our local health department through the WIC (Women, Infant, and Children) Supplemental Program. I worked there for about a year, and still stay in contact with the staff in case there is any assistance I can provide.

My journey with my first-born started in 2002, when I never saw breastfeeding in my everyday life, and now I see breastfeeding every-where! Better still, I am proud to say that breastfeeding has become a "norm" in my family. All the women who have given birth since my second baby was born in 2007 have initiated breastfeeding. Knowing I made a positive impact on them brings me great joy, and while their breastfeeding experiences have all been different and varied in length, I know that even one day of breastfeeding can make a difference to a new baby. Additionally, my African American friends and associates have sought me out for assistance, a very powerful realization for me: I am assisting in "the movement."

My breastfeeding success wouldn't have been possible without loving support from my husband and my online friends. My advice for pregnant women is to choose the way they like to communicate: face to face, talking over the phone, texting, emailing, or chatting via social media, and seek out those types of resources to learn as much as possible. As you learn you will become empowered and your empowerment will lead to success, no matter what your breastfeeding goal may be.

Chapter 3

 # Pumping and Working

The majority of households are dual-income these days, and approximately two-thirds of women work outside of the home. Breastfeeding mothers who fall into this category must find a way to work and pump their breastmilk so that their babies can be fed while they are apart. Breastfeeding while working can be stressful, at least in the beginning. As with anything that is new and unknown, breastfeeding and pumping while working can take time to figure out. A mother's concerns may include when to introduce a bottle to her baby, which bottle to use, how much milk her baby will need when they are apart, where and when she will pump at work, and where she will store her milk. Unfortunately, not all employers support breastfeeding mothers, and not all women work jobs that make it easy to stay on a pumping schedule. Awareness regarding breastfeeding in the workplace is increasing, as is the Federal government's support of breastfeeding with income-tax incentives for breast pumps and supplies, as well as mandated insurance coverage for these items and professional lactation care (Internal Revenue Service, 2011).

Many employed women know where to turn for help, having sought help online during their pregnancies. There are Yahoo! groups, Facebook pages, and entire websites dedicated to supporting breastfeeding mothers in the workplace. In addition to the many breast-pump choices and their *accoutrements*, there are hands-free pumping bras, nursing covers, special milk-storage coolers, adapters for breast pumps to permit milk expression while riding in the car, and door hangers to let people know you'd like privacy while you are expressing that liquid gold!

Working and pumping takes commitment and willingness to figure out what works best. Some who have never faced these challenges may think that they are no big deal. But just ask any mother who has left her baby in the care of someone else while she resumed her duties on the job while continuing to breastfeed, and she'll tell you a different story. Melissa Perry, a mother who has breastfed all three of her children while working says:

> I still stand by the thought that while breastfeeding is best, you cannot argue that for a mother working outside the home, it is more convenient than formula-feeding. To nurse a child and work full time outside the home takes a lot of commitment, time, and energy. You have to pump on schedule every day or risk losing supply. You have to find a space to do it in, and in most cases for me, that space was a bathroom. You spend lots of money finding a pump to get it done quickly and efficiently, then you have to store the milk once you've expressed it—and that's just the logistical part. There are still the issues you face with supply, letting down for the pump, etc. Breastfeeding rocks if you stay at home, bar none, but it's really hard for someone who works outside the home.

Breastfeeding mothers who work outside of the home should know that there are valuable resources and a seemingly endless supply of mothers waiting to help, encourage, and support them as they work to meet their breastfeeding goals.

Monica's Story

My background of breastfeeding before having my daughter was limited. I grew up knowing my younger brother was breastfed, and I found out, while pregnant, that I was also breastfed. I do not remember growing up around nursing. Heck, I don't even remember my mother talking about it either. My mother breastfed me until I was nine months old, and my brother until he was 14 months old. Her only resource was her older sister who was always doing the "hippie" thing in the 1970s. My mother has said that if it weren't for her sister, she would have never breastfed. She had a positive role model for nursing.

40

Thirty years later, I found myself pregnant and had no idea where to begin "learning" how to breastfeed. So I went to the Internet, and started with the only thing I had ever heard of, the *What to Expect While Expecting* website, and then turned to Babycenter.com. After reading a few forums on these websites, I felt they weren't the best fit for me, so I kept searching. During my pregnancy, I subscribed to various gentle-parenting groups and pro-breastfeeding Facebook groups; looked for new moms on Meetup.com; and signed up for a new-mother La Leche League breastfeeding class. I always knew that I was going to breastfeed; I honestly never thought of the alternative. Looking back, I understand that this line of thinking might have set me up for failure in the beginning if we had not had such a great start.

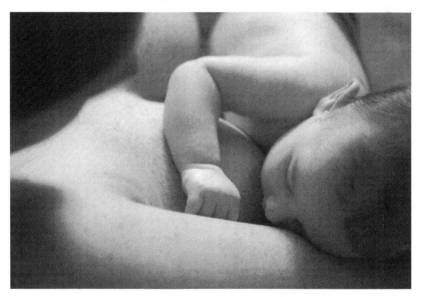

Monica with Zoe, enjoying newborn skin-to-skin time, before pumping on the road became the new norm for her as a working mom. — *Photo Credit: Sara McClure*

The first thing I knew that would help me with a successful breast-feeding relationship was to have an all-natural, drug-free birth. After all the research I had done online, to me, this was the first step in successful breastfeeding. I gave birth at a hospital with an obstetrician who also had a drug-free birth and allowed her breastfed children to self-wean. Due to some high-risk health issues during my pregnancy, it made sense to give birth in a hospital. Thankfully, I had the birth that I wanted and no real complications. My daughter was given to me immediately for skin-to-skin contact, and I nursed her within 15 minutes of her birth. During my stay at the hospital, I never put her down. She was held every moment by me. She slept in my arms, and I basically kept her at my breast at all times. I requested a lactation consultant at the hospital, and the one I met was helpful, teaching me positioning—specifically, the football hold—as my daughter was congested and this helped her nurse better.

Early on, I had an easy breastfeeding relationship with my daughter, but like any relationship, you have many highs and lows. I turned to my online groups right before I went back to work after being off for ten weeks. Like many mothers returning to work, my anxiety level was high, and I was obsessed with building up a stash before I returned to work. I found everything from "how to store breast milk" videos on YouTube, online checklists for returning to work, and an evening La Leche League meeting for working moms. I am a full-time working mom whose work situation is a little different in the fact that I am in sales, and my "office" is my car. So, returning to work brought two challenges for me: learning how to pump, and pumping on the road in my car. Once again I turned to online groups and resources to try and come up with a mobile pumping system.

After more than a year of pumping on the road, I only had a few incidents that made me break down and start crying. One day I was parked at a gas station in the middle of "Nowhere," Texas. I pulled into the back corner of the gas station to set up to pump, much like any other day. I was about an hour overdue to pump, so I was quite engorged and leaking. I still had one more appointment left for the day, and there was no way I could put off expressing milk any longer! I set everything up on the pump, got all situated, and just then, the motor on my pump quit working. I looked at my boobs, and thought "well I guess I am doing this manually." I pulled the right one out, started manual breast compressions, and right then a truck driver walked up to my car. He pulled back quickly, and apologized embarrassed. I never found out why he was walking up to my car, but I bet I gave him an eyeful!

All the places I have pumped while on the road: gas stations, airports, carwashes, many of my customers' companies' "mothers' rooms," my car, parks, grocery stores, the courthouse, and pumping while driving (while I never wanted to do this, it did happen a few times). I often thought "Pumping While Driving" should have been the name of my blog!

I've found that connecting online with other mothers who are going through the exact same thing you are going through helps tremendously. I feel like online moms are way more honest with what is going on with their children. Often, you get a group of mothers together for a play date, and they tend to exaggerate how well things are going with their children. Online mom groups tend to be more real or open, as they are usually there for the same reason: they need support.

Courtney's Story

I come from a family who breastfeeds. My mother breastfed all four of her children (with me breastfeeding the longest—until I was 15 months old), my aunt breastfed my cousin for a year, and my older sister breastfed her children for a year. Breastfeeding to a year is normal and expected, and like the other women in my family, a year was my initial goal.

When pregnant with my oldest son, my husband and I took Bradley Method Birthing Classes. Our instructor would nurse her 18-month-old during class sometimes when he acted restless. It was a bit uncomfortable at first for several of the parents-to-be, either because they had never witnessed any breastfeeding or witnessed breastfeeding by child over a year old. Over the course of 12 weeks while we were in class, it became less awkward and we could truly see that it was just a mother providing for her child. I still assumed that I would breastfeed for a year, though.

I gave birth in a hospital, and was in labor a total of 45 long hours. At 40 hours, I received an epidural, which I had a bad reaction to, and as a result was unable to hold my son for about three hours after his birth. By then, it was midnight, we were all exhausted, and breast-feeding just wasn't happening with exhausted parents and baby. The following morning, we made several attempts to breastfeed with little success. His latch was shallow, and I couldn't get in a comfortable position. Awkward to say the least. Finally at about 2 o'clock in the afternoon, my son latched on with the help of a nipple shield, and was able to nurse for a little while. (In hindsight, we did not need the nipple shield, and it was terrible to get him weaned from that). He nursed a few more times at the hospital before we went home.

The first night home, we all just slept. I woke up in a panic about 6 a.m., but all was well: just a sleepy baby! With the use of a nursing pillow, I was able to get my son into a more comfortable position, but we continued to struggle. For three weeks, it was very difficult, painful (even with the shield), and frustrating, but we stuck with it. My mom helped get him to latch better and offered a lot of encour-agement. Pretty soon, he was nursing like a pro and we finally got rid of the nipple shield.

I returned to work at ten weeks postpartum and managed to pump for 15 minutes, three times a day while at work. Luckily, I never had a real production issue (I thought I did a few times, but it was just supply adjusting accordingly and never caused any issues). I thought I would pump for a year, just like I would breastfeed for a year.

Shortly after returning to work, on one of my many pumping breaks, I was searching online for information about supply issues and came across the CafeMom website (www.cafemom.com). Seeking to feel more connected to other moms who had children the same age, I signed up. I found many helpful groups on this site, and the breastfeeding group is one of my favorites. The women in this group helped me overcome fears that my supply was failing, gave tips for my first business trips away from my son, and other wonderfully reassur-ing advice. From this group of women and others, I learned about full-term breastfeeding and the importance of full-term breastfeeding for both mother and baby.

After becoming a member of CafeMom, I went on to follow many blogs and groups on Facebook that dealt with natural parenting and attachment parenting styles. Being a full-time working mother, the time spent with my son is so important to me. I spend time every day on CafeMom now. I am now one of the more veteran breastfeeding moms who can offer support and advice to others. I have also continued to rely on support and advice from mothers who have many more years of experience than I have, especially as I enter new territory.

My son is now 29 months old, and still nursing. I pumped at work until he was 18 months and had enough milk stored that he received breast milk at daycare until he was two. The newest chapter in my life is tandem breastfeeding! I am currently 30 weeks pregnant, and have nursed the whole pregnancy. My current plan is to tandem nurse once his baby brother arrives.

Without the support I found online, I'm not sure that I would have had the courage to do what felt right to me (full-term breastfeeding and attachment parenting). It is reassuring to know that I am not alone and my choices are valid. The support from online forums not only enhanced my breastfeeding relationship, but my mothering skills as well. I will be forever grateful to the women who helped guide me to this path.

The most important advice for new mothers seeking online support is that not all information is accurate or good. Do not let anyone online bully you for your choices, whether they are full-term breastfeeding or early weaning. You are ultimately the person who makes decisions based on what is best for your family. And always do your research! The more educated you are before baby arrives, the better.

Alysia's Story

Breastfeeding is a passion of mine, but prior to becoming a mother, I was never exposed to it. I do not know if my brother or I were breastfed, as I never felt comfortable asking my mom questions about it. I didn't really know anything about parenthood, either, but I pictured all of my children sleeping peacefully through the night in cribs, tucked in their perfectly decorated nurseries, breastfeeding during the day, eventually giving them jarred baby food, all while wearing a shift dress with matching pumps, a pearl necklace, and a smile on my face! Little did I know what parenthood would actually look like. A divorce, remarriage, co-sleeping, baby-led weaning, extended nursing, baby wearing, toys strewn everywhere, piles of laundry on the changing table (that's where the clean clothes come from), one kid sleeping in our bed, one in a crib in her room, and the other sleeping in his bed or sometimes on the couch, and I'm lucky I get out the door to go anywhere on time, let alone with matching shoes!

All three of my children were born in hospitals. My oldest is my ten-year-old son, and when he was born there was no Facebook, and no such thing as a smart phone. I always dreamed of being a stay-at-home mom, like my mom was. She seemed happy doing it, so I

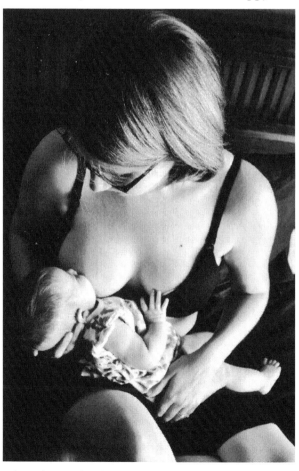

Alysia breastfeeding her daughter. — *Photo credit: Jessica Bekowitz*

thought I would be happy doing it as well. After I gave birth to my son, I had to have a D&C for a retained placenta. I didn't have a birth plan or a breastfeeding plan, and while I was under anesthesia undergoing my procedure (less than two hours), the nurses gave him his first bottle. I stayed in the hospital for three days, and he did not nurse well for any of those days. There was no lactation consultant on staff, and the nurse just held him up to my boob while he screamed. It was not a positive experience, and was quite uncomfortable and scary. We got home and my milk came in, but it was a forceful letdown, and it choked him. I never thought to turn to the Internet for help. I read in my book, *What to Expect When You're Expecting*, and it said the baby should latch on, and had an archaic looking drawing of a mother and infant bonding while nursing. I wanted to scream at the book, and rip the pages out and throw them in the fireplace. Was it because something was wrong with my boobs? Was it because he got a bottle at the hospital? Why, why, WHY? I had no answers and no help.

You know what else wasn't widely discussed ten years ago? Postpartum depression (PPD) and obsessive-compulsive disorder (OCD). Six years later, I realized that I had a severe case of PPD; I struggled with depression and OCD before having children, and stopped my medication when I was pregnant. I didn't want to take any medication while nursing, but I was a mess. I was a stay-at-home mom like I always wanted, with this beautiful baby boy, and all I could do was lie around in my pajamas and cry all day. I remember lying on the bed, crying with my son because I didn't know what was wrong with him. Eventually, I realized that staying home was not for me, and I went back to work. But those were two of the darkest years of my life.

Five weeks after having the baby and struggling with nursing, I was bawling in the office of the pediatrician. She said he wasn't gaining weight fast enough, and I should stop trying to breastfeed and start giving him formula. "It's okay," she said, "They wouldn't make formula if it wasn't good for babies." I was devastated, but someone with a medical degree was telling me this wasn't working. I was a community-college dropout, so I figured she must be right. I stopped nursing, and started giving him formula. And I've never stopped having guilt about it. He had ear infections every month for two years, and I always blamed myself. Even now that he's ten, healthy, and too smart for his own good, I could still have a good sob fest about it if I let myself dwell for too long on it.

Eight years later, I had my first daughter. I was *determined* to breastfeed this child. I had no complications after childbirth, but just in case, I told everyone with whom we came in contact that she was not to have a bottle. I'm certain the hospital staff probably referred to me as "That Annoying Girl In Room 203 Who Won't Shut Up About Breastfeeding Her Baby." I don't know what I did differently, but I was able to breastfeed her. She was always sleepy, so my biggest struggle was keeping her awake to nurse. It was frustrating at times, but we persevered. Sadly, there was still no support offered to me by the hospital. I was there for two nights, and a lactation consultant never visited me. I had not yet found an active support group, online or otherwise, although I was better-versed on the Internet, and I had found the KellyMom website and other sites related to pumping. I didn't have any postpartum depression issues after giving birth, and I felt encouraged by that.

Since I wasn't a stay-at-home mom anymore, I was going to pump when I went back to work from maternity leave. I started "practicing" my pumping schedule the week before I went back to work. I loved how easy it was to pump. I didn't have to struggle with nursing when she was really tired, and my husband could help feed her (his nickname amongst my friends is "Mr. Perfect"). So I quit nursing; and when she was about six months of age, I regretted that decision. I went somewhere and forgot my pump. I had brought enough breast milk with me, so the baby was fine, but my breasts were engorged and I was in a lot of pain at the end of that day. I tried to nurse her, but she pushed my breast away, not recognizing it as a food source. I was crushed that day, but overall, I felt successful. My daughter was getting what I felt was best for her.

I pumped until she was ten months old, and then I found out I was pregnant with my third child. My daughter had been a high-risk pregnancy, so I immediately stopped pumping, since I knew that nipple stimulation could cause contractions. I had enough milk stored so that she could have bottles until almost one year old. We did have to supplement with formula the last month, but I felt like I did the best I could.

When my third baby was born, another little girl, I was determined to breastfeed, and this time, I was committed to pumping and feeding from the breast. Success again! After she was born, I only stayed in the hospital one night, and this time I was visited by a lactation consultant. By this time, though, I was an old pro. This little one isn't much of a sleeper, so trying to keep her awake was never an issue. She always latched right away, and she transitioned to bottles without a problem when I went back to work. She nurses like a champion when I get home from work. I think she misses it, because even if she has just had a bottle, as soon as I walk in the room, she goes straight for the boob! It makes me smile. My postpartum depression returned after she was born, but because of my history, I feel like I am able to manage it.

Right now, my goal is to pump and nurse for at least two years, and then see how things will go. Mr. Perfect is supportive of our current pumping/nursing situation. He says he is supportive of the extended nursing, then he adds the "but," which we all know is not supportive. The "but" is that he thinks extended nursing is "weird." I think he pictures our two-year-old nursing like an infant does; every two hours, and possibly in public. But our two year old has one bottle in the morning, more if she has a cold (I slip some of my pumped milk in with the regular milk), or an "ouchie." I picture it more like that. It's going to be a supplement to her three meals a day. It's going to soothe her when she falls down, or when she has a bad dream. I think once he sees what the reality of extended nursing looks like, he will actually be supportive.

I must confess that I used to relate participating in online groups with being a nerd, as the only exposure I had to them prior to looking for breastfeeding help, was from my ex-husband, who liked "Star Wars" message boards. I am aware now that message boards can be useful, and aren't just for fun. While I was pregnant with my second child, I was put on bed rest. I was bored out of my mind, and sought companionship on BabyCenter (www.babycenter.com). It was here that I found my first online-support group. A small group of women there formed a separate Facebook group, and I was hooked.

Eventually, I engaged in a few other Facebook groups; one for pregnancy, another for breastfeeding support, and finally one for post-partum depression. In these groups, I learned all about what other women were going through—what was "normal," what foods would increase my supply, what was common in other cultures. They helped me get through mastitis with my third child. I had support, not only when breastfeeding went wrong, but also when life went wrong. I was also able to contribute my experience, I felt valued. Having found it odd to bond with "strangers," I laugh now because I consider these women my sisters, people I trust with intimate details of my life. We talk in our groups every single day. I still rely on these groups to help with baby questions (you still have questions even after having three children), breastfeeding questions, parenting questions, sex questions, menstrual-cycle questions, etc. No subject is off limits.

What is the difference between where I started and where I ended up? I'm not sure if I will ever have an answer to that. Was it what I ate during pregnancy? Was it the relationships I was in at the time? Was it the drugs I had during childbirth? Was it the depression? Was it the information I found online? Was it the community-online sup-port? The world may never know. I know that I will never be able to shed the mommy guilt that I have from not breastfeeding my son. What I do know is that the importance of breastfeeding my other two children may not have been as great if not for that experi-ence, so for that I am thankful.

I would encourage any woman who is pregnant, or considering getting pregnant, to find an online-support group. You can find a wealth of knowledge, experience, and support for nearly anything that you are going through. You will never feel alone in your expe-rience. I will caution you against doing anything that makes you uncomfortable. Just because someone had an experience similar to yours, and had a certain solution and positive outcome, doesn't mean that's the only path. You still have your values, your thoughts, your gut feeling. Take bits and pieces of what everyone shares with you, mold it, and shape it into what works best for you and your family.

Chapter 4

A Mother's Loss: Breastfeeding After Losing a Child

The love we feel for our children connects us to other women. Becoming a mother means you view the world in a new way, and you feel it much more deeply. We often joke about how just one Hallmark-card commercial can leave us in tears on the couch, and there is a really good reason for that. Major physical changes occur during pregnancy and childbirth: ones that literally make us different people. There have been recent studies on fetal microchimerism, the transmission of cells from mother to child and vice versa, and these cells have been shown to linger in mothers' bodies for decades. Add to this the chemical connection that breastfeeding creates, the hormone oxytocin being released from skin-to-skin contact, and you realize that there is another facet of motherhood that is almost beyond our reach. We can't change or expel the cells our babies leave behind in our bodies, just as we can't stop the flood of oxytocin into our blood when our babies latch on to feed. These physical changes help us bond emotionally to our babies. Before we know it, things that never moved us before can leave us grabbing for the nearest box of tissues.

I remember when I became a mother, I'd look at adults and suddenly wonder what they were like as babies. It was almost as if I had to reinterpret the world now that I had a baby of my own. Sometimes, when he was just a tiny newborn, I would hold my oldest son and have the most vivid daydreams about disasters happening, and almost panicking because I had no idea how I would ever save him in such an event. I used to tell these strange fantasies to my husband, and it was clear he couldn't relate. When I told my sister, she said, yes, that it was normal and many mothers do it. If you ask a mother what her worst fear is, she will respond—losing my child. Sadly mothers are faced with losing their children, and when it happens, it's devastating. I mentioned that my husband couldn't relate to my weird fantasies about disasters, and I think that sometimes the same can be said when mothers go through infant loss. They need to connect to other women. Perhaps it is because we understand the "layer of motherhood" that is beyond our reach and lies deep in our physiology? The emotional support women offer each other is different than that offered by men—not better, just different. When deep grief strikes after the tragic loss of a child, having a group of sisters to lean on can be crucial in helping deal with the situation.

Many of the stories in this book are from women who don't know one another, but Joanna and JoEllen are different. They actually met online and their friendship blossomed long before tragedy struck, when their greatest bond was the common practice of breastfeeding. Years later, their friendship strengthened in a way they could have never expected, when they turned to one another for emotional support as they each worked through the grief of losing their babies.

Joanna's Story

Before I had children, I knew that I wanted to breastfeed. When I was pregnant with my first daughter, I knew that the state where I lived didn't, and still doesn't have much support for breastfeeding moms. So after doing some online research, I joined the online forum group on the La Leche League International website.

Almost six years and three children later, I can say that this community of moms has been amazing, not only to help me learn about nursing and to coach me through the difficult patches I had, but they have also been supportive for parenting tips and through trials that come with motherhood.

When I was pregnant with my first daughter, I knew that I would have to work during her first year. So many women in my everyday life made it sound like it was impossible to breastfeed and work, especially the pumping part of it, and that I would have to supplement with formula. Formula was not an option for me. I wanted to nurse my daughter and pump, feeding her my milk exclusively. For several months before she was born, I talked to lots of other moms on the

Mother-to-Mother forum, and they were amazing. I not only learned about how other moms had successfully nursed and pumped for their children, but they also gave me the support to hold to my values, even in the midst of people telling me I couldn't. When Alayna was born, nursing started off well. I didn't have any problems with supply or latching, but I did end up having a traumatic birth. I had a c-section, and while there are some cases where a c-section is necessary, mine was not. At this point in my mothering journey, my online community helped me not only with nursing my daughter, but gave me support while I recovered from a very traumatic birth experience. It was amazing to talk with other women who had suffered traumatic births and hear stories of their healing.

When I went back to work, my community of moms was so supportive and helped me with my pumping questions. I can honestly say that I didn't have a problem pumping. I believe that nursing and pumping can successfully be done when you have the emotional support you need, and these ladies were my support. There were working moms who encouraged me on those days that I was utterly exhausted and just wanted to stay home with my daughter, and there were other moms who gave me tips on how to get my milk to let down while at work by simply bringing with me one of my daughter's pictures and a blanket to hold. The first time I spilled my "liquid gold," these ladies understood how disappointing and upsetting it was. When I needed tips on how to store breast milk in the refrigerator and deep freezer, they told me how to do it! I believe that the majority of my success in working full time, breastfeeding, and pumping was due to the support of these women. They rallied around me.

Not only is breastfeeding challenging in the beginning, but being a first-time mom can be hard too. When I had questions about teething, or Alayna's sleep pattern, her nursing, or what type of foods to introduce, the LLLI forums were my go-to group of mothers. I remember one night Alayna had a rash, and my husband and I didn't know what to do. I turned to him and said, "I'm going to post something on the forums. Honey, these ladies will get back to me within the hour," and sure enough I had answers within 15 minutes! It was not only comforting, but reassuring to have women who were similar in parenting styles and values, and from whom I could glean advice.

I remember thinking that I would only nurse a year before I had Alayna. I had never known anyone to nurse over a year. I quit my job when Alayna turned one, and no longer needed to pump. Thankfully, my online mamas taught me about the benefits of nursing past one year of age. I didn't know how long I was going to nurse, but they encouraged and informed me that regardless of what people around me were saying, there was much evidence to support the continuation of our nursing relationship. I was able to make my own choice. These women not only supported me in listening to my questions and fears, I had a safe place to put it all out there where I knew I would not be judged.

While nursing Alayna, we lost a baby in the first trimester of pregnancy, and the LLLI community helped me through this time as well. When we found out we were pregnant, they reassured me that it was okay to nurse while pregnant, and gave me tips on how to do it, and encouragement along the way. When we lost our baby, this group also gave me the support I needed while I grieved, and showed me the research to let me know that the miscarriage was not caused by nursing. (Unfortunately, there were several people in my life who didn't know anything about nursing who implied that it was my fault—that if I weaned Alayna this would never have happened). My online friends offered support and education about how men and women grieve differently. They gave their own stories of miscarriage and how they individually dealt with loss. Although everyone grieves differently, it was so comforting to be around other women who were comfortable talking about their babies who have passed away in only the first trimester.

The next time I became pregnant, the LLLI online community not only helped me emotionally with being pregnant after a miscarriage and the fears I had of giving birth after a c-section, but they also helped me learn about tandem nursing. These ladies, through their own stories, gave me the courage to have a vaginal birth after cesarean (VBAC). Even when the doctors were telling me I couldn't do it, these ladies encouraged me that I could. They were my cheerleaders. I remember other women courageously sharing their stories with me of their successful VBACs, and assuring me up until the day I went into labor that I could do this. They helped me find resources that taught me which questions to ask, and to believe in myself. My successful VBAC with my second daughter Gwendolyn led me to tandem nurse Alayna and Gwendolyn for 11 months!

If not for this group of women, I don't know if I would have successfully tandem nursed. They helped me navigate those waters, and figure out how I could be comfortable nursing and tandem nursing in public—a personal success for me. I was discreet, but I was no longer concerned about what people thought, because I was equipped with the knowledge of why tandem and extended breastfeeding is so beneficial. So when people asked or looked, I politely and joyfully talked with them about the facts. Years later, I have moms come up to me and say that when they saw me tandem nursing or breastfeeding my toddler, it was such an encouragement to them to see my confidence.

I enjoyed nursing Alayna for three and a half years, and near the end I remember wondering, "how will I know when it's time to wean?" I of course asked my forum moms and they shared stories of how they knew, which was reassuring and helpful. The day I realized I was ready to wean, I was singing to Alayna at night, our usual routine, and she looked up at me and said, "Mommy, why did you sing so fast?" I needed her to interpret that sign for me, and once she did, I knew it meant I was ready to wean. It was the support that I got from this forum that gave me the confidence to know that we would recognize the moment.

When we became pregnant with our third daughter, Lydia Ann, I hadn't been online with my group in a little while, since I felt comfortable nursing, nursing while pregnant, tandem nursing, pumping, and weaning, but I still checked in from time to time. At our five-month ultrasound we learned that there was no hope for our daughter's survival. The LLLI online community was a major support for my family. These women embraced us while I carried our daughter. This online community provided me with a safe place to voice my grief.

It was also a place where tragedy was no stranger. I found several other moms who had lost their children at birth, or shortly after birth. Although none of us had gone through the same exact situ-

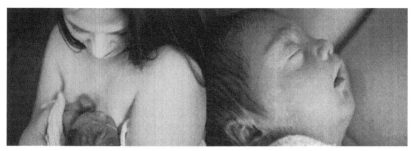

Joanna and newborn Lydia Ann bonding through breastfeeding and skin-to-skin. —*Photo credit: Stephanie Lyell*

ation, we had something in common. These women offered their support to me once more.

When Lydia Ann was born, she survived birth. The LLLI online community rallied around me once again, helping me to learn ways how to make my milk come in quickly for my baby who was medically fragile. I remember feeling very overwhelmed at the time. We had been told there was no hope for survival, and here she was breathing. She was three weeks early and weak. I tried to nurse her, but her suck was just so weak. When we got home the next day from the hospital, I was feeling very stressed and knew from the LLLI community that stress did not help anything when it came to your milk coming in. That afternoon, as I was pumping, I remembered hearing stories of woman on the forum who had used donated breast milk for their children. Thankfully, I had several lactating friends. I called one of them, and they brought over some frozen breast milk for me to use with Lydia Ann. Once that bottle was heated and my daughter was fed, my milk came in. There was something so relieving for me the moment I gave my daughter breast milk, and it didn't even have to be mine. I am so thankful to the women on the forum who shared their stories about donor milk.

During Lydia Ann's life, I regularly offered her to nurse at my breast, and while she suckled, she did not have strength to draw out the milk from my breast. The forum became another source of support during this time for me. I had experience pumping and working, but I had never been in a situation where the majority of my milk was being drawn out by a pump. These women once again helped me during this time. Through their encouragement and shared personal experiences, I was able to persevere and find a rhythm with pumping full time, while offering Lydia Ann the breast regularly.

Lydia Ann passed away when she was 27 days old, and my friends supported me, to help me transition from nursing a newborn to solely nursing my almost two year old. They helped me know what to do with engorgement. They gave me tips on what to do at my daughter's visitation, and funeral in case I experienced my milk letting down while there. I remember one of my friends from LLLI came to my daughter's visitation to represent the community. I cannot fully put into words what it felt like to see her there, representing these women from across the country who had walked the journey with us through Lydia Ann's life and death.

I know that this is supposed to be about breastfeeding support, but I have to say that while I joined this community for just that, I received so much more. Not only did I have cheerleaders to help me meet my breastfeeding goals and women who were well-versed on breastfeeding and able to send me links to the research, I had a community of moms who supported me through the death of two of my children, and who tangibly helped our family in the aftermath of Lydia Ann's death. Almost a year later, this community continues to be a source of support through grief.

I believe that breastfeeding is one of the most important choices I have ever made in my life as a mother. I believe that I was able to achieve my own personal goals because of the support of this online community. I believe that not only did this community give me the knowledge and support I needed to breastfeed all three of my children, they have helped me grow into the mom I am today. Being a mom is hard. Breastfeeding is challenging. We as moms need support, and these women have supported me the last six years in more ways than I could ever imagine.

JoEllen's Story

I sought support for breastfeeding online in early 2008 when my oldest son, my first child, was about one month old. At the time, I had been lurking on a message board and soon noted how divisive it was. In their signatures, mothers would proclaim a series of parenting choices:

> *Co-sleeping, non-vaxing, cloth-diapering, PROUD*
> *attachment parenting, extended-breastfeeding mama!*
> *Formula-feeding mom to two girls. We love our Pampers!*

I had no idea why anyone felt the need to make such declarations. I wasn't so sure what attachment parenting (AP) was either, but after Googling for a bit, decided that it sounded an awful lot like what we were doing. The AP moms on that message board were few in number, and quite defensive in any given thread. Thus began the search for a new online hangout.

I joined the La Leche League International (LLLI) Mother-to-Mother forums soon after. So-called "crunchy moms" were well-received there, but the forums were not exclusive to those. "Take what you need and leave the rest," was the motto. I was greeted with encouragement and relevant information. Logan and I powered through our early struggles, and with the support of the ladies on the forums, we enjoyed breastfeeding until he weaned at two years. When he was a newborn I said that I would only nurse him for a year, but that quickly changed! Breastfeeding for a longer duration than I had witnessed in real life had become normal to me.

As time passed, my friendships grew and strengthened. I gave support to the other ladies as often as I received it. We offered virtual shoulders to cry on in times of joy and loss. This was never truer for me personally until June 2011.

I became pregnant with Lincoln, my second son, after a long season of multiple miscarriages. We embarked on his pregnancy with great hope. I had learned a great deal about normal birth, and how modern birthing practices often negatively impact breastfeeding, as had been the case with my first. We decided to plan a homebirth for our second birth.

Lincoln's home-water birth was one of the most incredible experiences of my entire life. He was delicious, with thick, dark hair and deep, soulful eyes. He nursed well from the start! On his third day of life, he began to struggle with nursing. It became evident late that

58

night something was terribly wrong with more than breastfeeding. We took Lincoln to the emergency room, where he was soon transported downtown to Cincinnati Children's Hospital Medical Center. Lincoln was diagnosed with a critical congenital heart defect that had not shown up on the mid-pregnancy ultrasound. We were told that he had Hypoplastic Left Heart Syndrome, and had essentially been born with only half a heart.

The LLLI ladies sprang into action. While our family was encased in the thick fog of confusion and fear, the ladies rallied the troops. Within the first few days, an online fundraiser was set up to help alleviate the costs of us driving to the hospital each day, missing more work than planned, and whatever else. Cards came pouring in from across the country. Care packages arrived with practical items, as well as handmade gifts. Prayer chains were started in congregations of people we will most likely never meet.

Our Lincoln fought a hard battle for three months. He passed away in September 2011, while waiting for a heart transplant. The ladies lifted our family up during that time too. On the forums, I was free to pour out my pain and grief. I was able to smile and find joy there too. The ladies were never afraid to say Lincoln's name, or mention him in conversation the way that some people we interacted with in person were. At his memorial service, three of the ladies made the drive to be there for us. I will never forget that day.

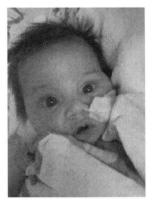

I expressed my desire to donate or share all of the milk I had pumped for Lincoln. The LLLI ladies knew better than anyone how much it meant for that milk to be used. To throw it away would have added another layer to our loss. I was connected with mothers from states far away who received my milk—all 3,000 ounces of it in total—with deep gratitude.

In December 2011, I discovered that I

Lincoln, with this thick hair and soulful eyes, after one of his breast-feeding sessions in the hospital with his mama, JoEllen. —*Photo credit: JoEllen Noble* was pregnant again, this time with our son Leonidas. I was a mental and emotional mess. The ladies never wavered in their encouragement and optimism. Along with us they cried and cheered. Leo was born one week before the one-year anniversary of Lincoln's passing. I think his birth was special for my dear friends too. Through the LLLI ladies, I experienced a depth of love I had not encountered before. They understood my tears of frustration from my trials to breastfeed, to my tears of the most unimaginable pain. The ladies have always stood by us. I know some might say that it is not possible to find true love online, but I did. I met my best friends there.

Chapter 5

Breastfeeding Preemies in the NICU

Ask any pregnant woman who is past her estimated due date what she wants most, and the chances are likely that she'll say something like, "to not be pregnant forever!" We joke about it at the end of a long 40 weeks of sharing our bodies, watching them change, longing for our old non-maternity clothes and toes that don't look like sausages—but we really just want healthy babies. If that means we endure a little extra time being pregnant and uncomfortable, we tend to forget about it once we look into our child's eyes for the first time.

Premature birth, that which occurs before a baby is 37 weeks gestation, can occur even if a mother does "everything right." The Centers for Disease Control and Prevention lists the following as risk factors for premature birth: carrying more than one baby (twins, triplets, or more); problems with the uterus or cervix; chronic health problems in the mother, such as high blood pressure, diabetes, or clotting disorders; certain infections during pregnancy; and cigarette smoking, alcohol use, or illicit drug use during pregnancy (Centers for Disease Control and Prevention [CDC], 2012). Nearly one out of every eight babies is born prematurely, so it is something that we should really be aware of; if you did not have a premature baby, you probably know someone who did. Premature babies usually spend time in Neonatal Intensive Care Units (NICUs), and the length of the stay depends on how early they were born and how medically fragile they are.

Breastfeeding is essential to help preemies grow and catch up to where they need to be. When a mother gives birth prematurely, her milk is specially designed to protect her baby and help him grow, a fascinating mechanism of milk-making and a woman's body. Motherhood ignites a certain amount of worry in all women; it's innate, it's instinct, and we can't turn it off.

When a woman gives birth to a premature baby, it can be an

extremely emotional time and her mental state may be just as delicate as her tiny baby. She has to accept that her pregnancy didn't go as she imagined, and she worries now because she is often separated from her baby, who must be cared for in the NICU. In addition, she still has all of the other stresses of everyday life to bear: work, other children and family, school, bills, etc. None of it stops just because she has a premature baby. It can be such a trying time in a mother's life, and support is crucial. Twenty years ago women with preemies couldn't reach out online and connect with other mothers who could understand their fears, nor was it as easy to access breastfeeding information that was specific to pre-term babies. Krysta and Kelly sought help online to guide them through their journeys with premature babies. Their emotional strength as mothers could stand strong against the fiercest of foes, and they both agree they couldn't have survived without an army of online moms supporting, encouraging, and educating them along the way.

Krysta's Story

I grew up with minimal exposure to breastfeeding. My youngest sibling, six years my junior, was breastfed until she was one year of age, but I also remember seeing pictures of my sister and me using a bottle. One of the family stories told is how I, as a toddler, would climb into my sister's crib to finish her bottle after she fell asleep. Another family story is how one time my eldest brother and a friend, about ten years old at the time, came into the house while our mom was nursing our youngest brother. The friend asked, "What is your mom *doing?*" "She's just feeding my *little brother*," my brother replied complete with an eye roll. I never saw a big deal one way or another and didn't really think about it.

My sister became pregnant before me and had a mild case of preeclampsia, which led her doctor to induce her. He ended up using forceps to deliver my niece, which bruised her face, and my sister was barely able to nurse at all as a result. When my husband and I decided to try getting pregnant, I was working as a graphic artist for a local paper, spending a lot of time bored and online. When pregnancy didn't come easily, I joined the Babycenter and the *What to Expect When You Are Expecting* online groups for women trying to conceive. After 11 months and fertility medications, we became pregnant.

Once I dove into my Babycenter-birth-month group, I really started see the mommy wars. I found out about the parenting-method debate, diaper debate, circumcision debate, vaccination debate, babywearing debate, and the breastfeeding debate. I joined more groups, began reading articles and blogs, and absorbed all of the information I could. Somehow, I found Best for Babes (www. BestforBabes.org) and The Leaky Boob (www.theleakyboob.com) breastfeeding resources. I kept randomly running into "preemie" things, but ignored them since I knew I would have a healthy full-term, vaginal delivery, where my baby would be put directly on my chest to nurse immediately.

Near the end of my second trimester, my husband and I decided to relocate for a career opportunity, and I let him leave ahead of me to handle the logistics while I stayed with my mother during the short two-month period we agreed upon. At 25 weeks, my fingers began to swell, and without giving it much thought I attributed it to normal pregnancy swelling. The next day, while putting that week's paper together, I had my legs propped up to try and help with the swelling. I had apparently been shifting my leg the against the knob of my desk drawer, because when I looked at them, there were dime-sized circles all over the side of my calf. I remembered indentations that failed to go away as being a sign of preeclampsia, so I called my sister, who worked in the same office, into my cubicle. She poked her finger in my leg, and it left at least a half-inch indentation. We called my doctor and our mother, and drove over an hour away to my doctor to check my blood pressure. I was just under the preeclampsia threshold, and I had also gained a great deal of weight overnight. My doctor sent us home with a 24-hour urine test, and strict instructions to take my blood pressure frequently. If it went over 150, I was to report to the hospital immediately.

The next morning my mother reminded me to take my blood pressure. It was 170/98, and half an hour later, it was 168/98. After a couple more attempts, we followed the doctor's advice, and drove in so I could be monitored. Once we arrived, I was admitted to Labor and Delivery for a few hours of observation, which led to an overnight stay. During this time I had an ultrasound. The tech was really quiet and asked me how sure I was about my due date. She also pointed out that my baby had a "clover heart," meaning the bottom two chambers of his heart appeared as one.

After she left, the doctor on call came in and grilled me on how sure I was about my due date. I finally yelled, "I'm sure. I was on Clomid! I know exactly when he was conceived!" To which he replied, "Ohhh, he is a Clomid baby! They always run small. He has been about a week behind on all his ultrasounds." and he left the room. The next morning my obstetrician came in right after church, still in her dress clothes and told me, "There is something wrong with his heart and he is measuring about four weeks too small." We immediately went into shock. No one had told us how small he was. I barely remember hearing her say, "I know how hard we worked to get this baby. If I were in your shoes, I would want to be in Jackson, so, I'm sending you to Jackson."

A few hours later, I was at the University Hospital in Jackson, and on magnesium. If you have never been on magnesium, it makes your body feel like you are in a parka on a 100 degree day, in the sun. I had a huge team of doctors. My son, however, had none, as I was informed by one of the doctors, "We are here for you, not him." The fetal specialist was on vacation. On the second day, my husband managed to get a plane ride back, and was with me from then on.

Every morning, I received ultrasounds, where they were checking his blood flow, and testing to see how high his chances were of surviving another 24 hours. There was always between three and six doctors in the room each time. My urine protein levels were also being constantly checked, to see how my liver was faring.

On Thursday night, when my blood pressure spiked into the 200s, the doctors put me on a higher dosage of magnesium. The next morning we went down for our daily ultrasound. While waiting, my husband and I were joking around when yet another doctor came in. He said, "Well, it looks like we shouldn't have any trouble keeping you pregnant until Monday when the fetal cardiology specialist will be back, and then he can get a good look at him!" He walked out of the room, only to return five minutes later. But this time the mood in the room changed. He sat down and said, "We just got your protein levels back. They have spiked. We have to deliver today. But since you're down here, we will go ahead and let you have your ultrasound." We immediately began calling my family. We had been told they would take me to deliver our son in an hour and a half, and my family was two hours away. They checked his blood flow again, and this time he failed. We were both heading toward a crash. There was no other way to look at it other than that he had to be delivered that day.

I had been told when I arrived at the hospital that a study had been done on 100 babies with his heart condition, which we now knew was called Tetralogy of Fallot (a.k.a., Blue-Baby Syndrome), who weighed less than 750 grams, and the survival rate past two weeks of age was zero. Our son weighed 590 grams (1lb 4oz). One doctor even suggested that it was foolish to have a c-section just so he would have a heartbeat, since he wasn't going to survive anyway. He had a 25% chance of surviving an induced vaginal delivery. I opted to give him the highest chance of survival I could.

Until this point I had been expecting that I was going to spend ten weeks on bed rest, so it was a bit of a shock to be told I would only be pregnant for a few more hours. Thankfully, some other cases were pushed ahead of me, and by the time I went back it was 7 o'clock p.m. My family had made it and shift change had happened. When my tiny son was handed to the catching nurse, and wrapped in a warm towel in the deafeningly silent operating room, she handed him off to a nurse practitioner that believed the "chances" don't matter. She believed that if he was fighting, we were going to fight too. She intubated him and rushed him to the NICU. When I finally got to the postpartum floor, I immediately requested a breast pump. I remembered from the random preemie info I had gathered that breast milk was literally the difference in life and death for micro-preemies. I hopped online, chatted on The Leaky Boob's Facebook page and pumped. I collected drops of colostrum and sucked them into tiny 1cc syringes from the pump flanges. Thankfully, because

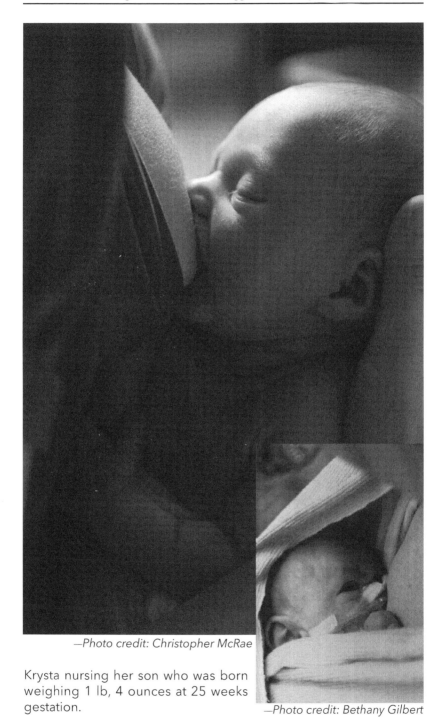

—*Photo credit: Christopher McRae*

Krysta nursing her son who was born
weighing 1 lb, 4 ounces at 25 weeks
gestation.

—*Photo credit: Bethany Gilbert*

of my time spent online, I knew that it was normal to receive such a small amount. My husband became the milkman and delivered the tiny syringes downstairs to our son's nurse every three hours.

I finally saw my son around 1 o'clock the next day. He was small and purple. He had such perfect little fingers and toes, and his head was about the size, shape, and feel of a perfectly ripe peach. I had to ask permission to touch him. I sat next to his humidified isolate until I needed more pain meds. Back in my room, I pumped some more and asked more questions online. I loved getting immediate feedback from those who had been there. When I was released days later, we moved to the Ronald McDonald House.

I pumped every three hours for the next month. I was getting ounces by then, but I was so tired that I nearly threw the pump through the wall. I couldn't look at the pump or think of my son, as so many pumping moms do when they pump, so I communed on Facebook and read. I also joined some other preemie groups, such as Breastmilk for Preemies (www.facebook.com/BreastmilkForPreemies) and Mended Little Hearts (www.mendedlittlehearts.org). It wasn't long before I was able to give advice to other preemie or pumping moms.

When my son was five months old, we were able to try and latch for the first time. It didn't work out so well. I was so scared that it wouldn't work, that it kind of became a self-fulfilling prophecy. The next day when I attempted again, I had chatted online with other moms about it and was much calmer. We were able to get him to latch, and he started nursing like a pro. Thanks to information from online moms, I knew to try nursing first. We even got the "but we want to use bottles so we know how much he is getting" from his resident. We did try some bottles so the nurses could bottle-feed him. We tried suggestions from moms. But due to his heart condition, combined with the weak lungs, we could only get one brand to kind of work. Even with that one it took 45 minutes for 20 cc (or less than an oz).

Before he was slated to go home, the neonatologists decided to check my calorie output, so they would know how to supplement his diet so he was getting the calories they wanted. When the test came back, the neonatologist's jaw nearly hit the floor, and she began begging me to donate, which I was unable to do due to postpartum depression medication I was taking. What did the test show? My body was producing milk that had 31.5 calories per ounce, which meant I could stop all fortifier packets that increased the calories in my son's diet. Due to our success, and his unexpected survival, our neonatologist was finally able to convince the hospital to get donor milk and only use human milk with all the micro-preemies. Through information posted online by one of my groups, I was able to show my doctor research on the benefits of nursing in the first 90 minutes. He loved the idea and ran with it. When I gave birth to my second child, I was able to nurse her within 30 minutes, and now the hospital uses this information for other mothers.

I still gleaned more information from the Internet after my daughter's birth—mostly about the first two months, since we missed that period with our son (three months early, five and a half months in the NICU). I had to learn what was "normal" for a breastfed newborn. At nearly three years old, we still rejoice anytime we are told something our son does is "normal." Our daughter still frequently shocks us at the things she does and learns on her own, long before we expect her to be able to do them.

I have calculated that I spent over 2,100 hours pumping during my son's NICU stay, and still prefer to be online when nursing my daughter. I ended up turning my blog into a NICU advice blog, and now have a page devoted to it. I have even written guest posts for another blog on how to breastfeed with a baby in the NICU. It would have been a much lonelier and more stressful experience had I not had social media to turn to—I was able to connect with other moms who "got it." It was the support I needed that no one in my "real" life could understand.

My sister and cousin also gained information to make nursing their second children successful through information I knew and things I reposted. I have also tried to encourage other moms to get into social media when it comes to breastfeeding, if for no other reason than to be able to get an immediate response to a question at 3 a.m.! I really love being able to be able to pay it forward, even if it is only through advice and links.

Kelly's Story

I gave birth to my first daughter, Cassidy, in the fall of 2008. I was induced at 38 weeks due to preeclampsia, and because of complications from previous surgery, my body couldn't dilate. The result was an emergency c-section at eight o'clock in the evening. Three hours later, we were reunited and I was able to nurse her immediately and, thankfully, without complications. She latched on and nursed like a champ! I knew when I was trying to get pregnant with my second daughter, that I wanted to nurse my next baby, and figured I wouldn't have any issues. I couldn't have been more wrong.

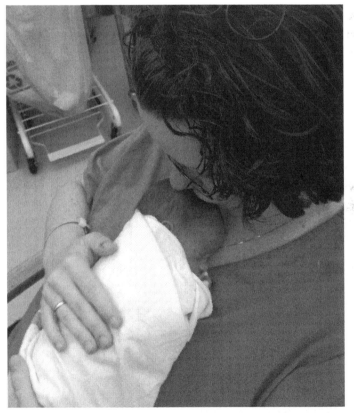

Kelly with her baby, Maggie, in the NICU. —*Photo credit: Kelly Boogertman*

When Cassidy was two and a half years old, my husband and I decided to try to get pregnant, and we were able to conceive as soon as we started trying! My second pregnancy was much easier, as with my first I had hyperemesis gravidarium (HG). I was lucky this time, and had no severe symptoms, and while I was nauseous a few times, I never got sick.

Unfortunately, I started showing the signs of preeclampsia again, earlier this time, at 31 weeks, and my obstetrician referred me to a high-risk specialist to be followed more closely. I received steroid injections to mature my baby's lungs, so that if it became necessary to deliver early she would be able to breathe on her own. Of course, we all agreed it was too early for her arrival.

At 33 weeks, I went for an appointment with my specialist, and when he took my blood pressure, it was very high: 180/110. The baby wasn't moving around well on the non-stress test, so they called the doctor who referred me to him. He sent me to Labor and Delivery for blood work. Of course, by this time I was an emotional wreck, and knew in my heart I'd be delivering her that day.

When I arrived at the hospital, my doctor did her best to calm me down and told me it would be fine, that they'd do the blood work, monitor me for a bit, and I'd go home. My husband arrived, my mother-in-law went home, and we waited.

My doctor came back in and told me that they were waiting for the one blood test, a liver panel, to come back so I could be released. At that point, I asked if I could use the bathroom. When my family helped me up, all we saw was the blood on the bed where I had been lying down. Having not experienced any bleeding during this pregnancy, I knew this was not a good sign. We immediately called my doctor. When I got to the toilet, I passed a very large blood clot and then I started bleeding profusely. I remember yelling, "Something just fell out of me, but it's not a baby!" and freaking out that I was making a mess on the bathroom floor. They got me back in bed and on the monitors, and did an ultrasound where they discovered that I was now having contractions. It was quickly determined that the bleeding was from the placenta. We waited a few minutes to see if the bleeding would stop, but it just kept getting worse. I later learned that I had a fourth-degree placental abruption, and I ended up losing over a quarter of my blood volume. Based on this diagnosis, they had no choice but to prepare me for a c-section. I sobbed because I knew 33 weeks was still too early, and I was so afraid for my baby.

They took me into surgery, gave me my spinal block, and started operating. My husband had called our parents, who were quite shaken and drove as quickly as possible to the hospital. The doctors wanted to lower my blood pressure, so they let me play with my iPhone in surgery; I literally "Facebooked" through my entire c-section operation.

Finally, I heard the tiniest, most pathetic little cry in the world; it sounded like a little kitten. I started sobbing again, and asked, "Is she okay?" Margaret Alice, or Maggie as we call her, made her debut weighing in at 3 pounds 5 ounces, and was 16 ¾ inches long. Soon though, her little kitten cry turned into a feisty little scream! They quickly brought her to my face so I could see her and kiss her. I had never seen anyone so small in my life. She was so beautiful, but also so very, very tiny. They whisked her away to the NICU, and finished up the surgery.

The next thing I remembered, I was in recovery and very weak. They were concerned that I was still bleeding. I didn't fully recognize yet why this was a concern, or how close I really came to not making it based on the amount of blood that I lost, and my brain wasn't able to comprehend how very dangerous the situation was. My mom, mother-in law, sister-in law, and aunt who is a NICU nurse at a neighboring hospital, came to see my little Maggie. They said she looked fantastic. Hearing that from a NICU nurse made me feel better, but I needed to see her. They promised they'd bring me to her before I went to my room. When they wheeled me in to her, I couldn't stop crying. She was on a CPAP machine, which they said was just for a little assistance in breathing, nothing serious was wrong. Once again, I was struck by how tiny she was. Finally, I got to my room, which to my dismay was a shared room. I was too tired to argue with the nurse who placed me there, but thankfully, I didn't have a roommate for the time being. As time went by, my husband and mother had to leave, and then I was alone.

I tried to sleep, but I was in so much pain and so scared. I found a friend online who was awake at 3 a.m., and asked her to call and talk to me and try to calm me down. She tried to calm me, but I was freaking out, it hurt so much. I called the nurse and she wouldn't give me anything. I immediately started having an anxiety attack. They couldn't calm me down, and the bleeding got a bit worse. They finally got a hold of my anesthesiologist, who yelled at them to give me some pain medication, which finally allowed me to get some much-needed rest.

In the morning, I had a new nurse, Judy, who I will always remember as my guardian angel. She called to check on my little one, who was perfectly okay. Judy brought me food, and even had the neonatologist to come up and speak to me since I was unable to leave. Unfortunately, when he came to see me, I had a second anxiety attack. I could not comprehend what he was saying to me, but I did give the hospital permission to put in an umbilical line for Maggie for added nutrition. I voiced my wish to breastfeed, and he said they'd wait to feed her until I could start pumping.

My anxiety refused to wane, and because my husband had to work, I called on my mother and all but demanded that she come to the hospital, telling her, "I just can't be alone any more!" When she arrived, my angel nurse Judy moved me to a private room, since she knew I couldn't have emotionally handled rooming with a mother who was able to have her healthy baby with her. Judy also took me to the NICU, where I ran into the neonatologist who had seen me during my anxiety attack. Because I hadn't held Maggie yet, she didn't feel *real* to me. I begged the doctor to let me hold her. The nurses were against it because of the CPAP, but the neonatologist told the nurses I wasn't going to get better without holding her. It was truly the happiest moment of my life knowing how sick I was and how small she was, and yet there we were.

It didn't last long, however, I started to get hot, dizzy, and nauseous. Judy appeared out of nowhere and took me upstairs, and then the non-stop vomiting began. It was eventually determined I had a gaseous bowel obstruction, and I began to wonder how much more my body would take. They had to insert an NG-tube while I was awake that went up my nose and down to my stomach, the worst experience ever, but it stopped the vomiting and allowed me to heal a bit. The next day, I felt much better, and they removed the tube and Judy helped me shower. I got down to the NICU, and Maggie was off her CPAP. I got to hold her and shower her with kisses and hugs, as did the grandparents, and my brother and his wife, but I wouldn't let anyone else hold her until my husband had his turn.

When I got back to my room, Judy brought in a breast pump and helped me start pumping. The nurses were ecstatic I was going to be breastfeeding, and told me how much better it was for the preemies. They called my milk "liquid gold." They gave me small bottles to pump into, and labels to mark the bottles as mine. The first night she was eating, they had to give her a teeny tiny bit of formula. After that, my milk came in fully and she was fed only that from then on.

By the time I left the hospital, I was freezing my milk because I was producing more than Maggie could eat. I was pumping every three hours, and soon had a full freezer of milk! Later, my supply dropped, and I of course panicked. I developed blisters on my nipples, which made me panic even more. Sadly, my health insurance company wouldn't cover a lactation consultant, or other professional breastfeeding help in the local area. A friend of mine, who was still nursing her three and a half year-old son, connected me with a group of mothers on Facebook who are all devoted to breastfeeding. They call themselves Modern Tribal Mamas (MTMs). I posted my plea for help, and immediately my inbox was flooded with recipes for lactation cookies, as well as information from lactation consultants who helped me realize my pump flanges were too small, and the blisters were from friction. These mothers helped me calm down, and were so helpful in those early days when I was so sick, so tired, running back and forth to the hospital, caring for a three-and-a-half-year-old who needed her mommy, and trying to heal. Maggie still wouldn't nurse as my nipples were just bigger than her tiny mouth. Once she came home, I continued to try, but she was so used to the bottle and wouldn't change.

Maggie never did nurse once she grew big enough. It was then that our pediatrician diagnosed her with tongue tie, but I didn't have the heart to have it snipped. She's already been through so much. However, each time I think I'm going to have to start supplementing with formula, the MTMs come through with new ideas, and I get back on track. Thanks to them, I still have some of my frozen stash from those early days when I needed back-up!

The mothers I met through Facebook have been extremely helpful with nursing and with other issues as well. A few weeks ago my breast pump motor died while I was pumping at work. Several mamas offered to bring a pump to me so I didn't have to go to buy a new one on my lunch break. Their remedies and suggestions have been so helpful and insightful every day, and I really rely on them more than I thought I possibly would. Surprising, since I've only met three of them in person, but I know all of them. They are my "tribe." They are my sounding board when I'm tired and she won't stop crying, or when I have any type of "mommy struggle." I find myself now offering advice to the moms who are new to the board, and giving out the recipe for lactation cookies, and all the advice they've given me to others.

For me, breastfeeding is hard. Anyone who says it isn't is lying or has a full-time maid and a cook. It's a sacrifice, especially when you're doing it my way, attached to a pump four to five times a day. I admit it: sometimes I feel like a dairy cow, but I know it's really the best thing for Maggie. Friends, and even family, told me in the beginning with Maggie I was nuts—that formula would get the weight on her quicker, but she gained weight quicker than any other baby in the NICU. Initially, they were adding a caloric fortifier to my milk, and they had to stop adding it because she was gaining weight so quickly. Even though Maggie came early, I still have her "due date" set as my goal: I want to pump until the one-year anniversary of it, and I am certain I will make it with a lot of help from my friends from Modern Tribal Mamas.

Chapter 6

Food Sensitivities

Breastfeeding is supposed to be easy, right? Your body does the work, and so long as you feed the baby regularly, the rest just takes care of itself! Well, not for all mothers—namely the mothers whose babies suffer from food sensitivities or allergies. These mothers can do everything "right" according to appearances: perfect positioning, good latch, cue feeding, etc., but it is the milk inside the breasts that poses the problem, not the act of breastfeeding itself. It is Extremely frustrating, and often depressing, to breastfeed a baby with food sensitivities. Trying to find the root of the problem can be an exhausting experience. Many newborn babies go through a normal fussy stage, and while frustrating for new parents because it can feel like trial by fire, it often subsides within a couple months. Before too long, the sometimes fussy, uncomfortable baby turns into one who coos and giggles, and parental heart-melting ensues!

For the mothers whose babies do have food sensitivities though, breastfeeding can be difficult. So what are some of the tell-tale signs? Fussiness, gassiness, skin rashes, nasal congestion, constipation or diarrhea (sometimes with blood present in the stool), and stubborn diaper rashes are among the most common. Mothers who notice these symptoms and suspect food allergies often start researching online before discussing the possibility of a problem with their doctors, lactation professionals, and family/friends with experience in this area.

The first step to solving the problem, if all signs point to a real probability of food-related issues, is for the mother to change her diet in an effort to eliminate offending foods. Elimination diets can be really hard. It's not only about having the willpower to avoid foods you enjoy. A baby with food sensitivities also requires you to find new foods to prepare to replace the old ones. Having to put mental effort into preparing new meals, avoiding much-loved foods, and keeping track of your baby's changes to these new dietary restrictions can be difficult, especially when added to the normal adjustment that all new mothers face.

When my oldest son was born, my step-mother came to visit and told me that some foods I was eating might be the cause of his fussiness. After paying careful attention to my diet I noticed that there seemed to be a connection between my diet and his temperament, specifically when I ate dairy. What was a new mother on a postpartum emotional roller coaster supposed to do without access to one of her favorite food groups? She sacrificed, and gave up the dairy. Motherly love won, and I did abstain from dairy for a few months. By the time I reintroduced it, he was okay with it and had outgrown his sensitivity.

It is, unfortunately, still the case that many healthcare providers receive no training about breastfeeding in medical school. As a result, they are often not knowledgeable about food sensitivities or allergies in breastfed babies, and many breastfeeding mothers can't get the answers and support about food sensitivities and allergies they need, so they go online for help. Mothers need a great deal of support when their babies have food allergies, because they need to know that they aren't failing, and that answers are out there—especially because their baby's health can be at stake. Having a baby who is struggling and doesn't feel well is stressful. Knowing that you are not alone, and that there are answers and others who can relate to the process can make all the difference to mothers who must travel this path.

Regina's Story

Our little boy Quinn was born after a fairly standard labor with a few snags here and there. Since my first child's labor and delivery was long and difficult, I was relieved to have this one be normal. Because we were Group B Strep positive, and I didn't realize how close I was to delivery when we headed to the hospital, we were required to stay 48 hours for labs and observation. This ended up being a blessing because it allowed me to simply rest and get to know my new baby boy without worrying about being at home or having our older child, a two-and-a-half-year-old girl, jumping on both of us.

The hospital's lactation counselor stopped by a few hours after birth, and after helping me remember how to hold a newborn to nurse, we were set and everything went smoothly. Quinn was efficient at nursing and seemed to love his milk comas. Since our first hardly slept at all from the day of her birth, I was thrilled to have a baby who actually slept. Quinn was a very content baby and I loved every quiet moment I had with him.

Somewhere around a week after birth, Quinn started breaking out in rashes, spitting up excessively and forcefully, having very runny and mucousy diapers, passing a significant amount of gas, appearing to be in intestinal distress, crying for long periods of time, developing patches of eczema all over his body, and becoming congested. The rash was especially severe on his bottom, where he developed blisters that broke open and bled. From experience with our first child, I knew that this was likely a food sensitivity we were dealing with. Since both my husband and daughter are sensitive to dairy, I eliminated dairy from my diet.

After a month, Quinn's symptoms had lessened in severity, but they weren't gone. He was gaining weight fine and meeting his milestones, but something was still bothering him. I turned to an online forum that I had found before our first child was conceived for help. The forum comprises many highly educated women, mothers, doctors, college professors, nurses—all of them very caring and willing to share their experiences to help others. I knew that many had dealt with food issues with their children and I trusted their advice. They had been encouraging me in the dairy elimination since it wasn't any easier than the first time I had done it for our daughter, and they knew we were struggling.

When I described Quinn's continued symptoms, I was met with a wide range of ideas. These ideas ranged from as severe as an inability to process proteins that would necessitate a special formula, to as simple as a yeast infection or bacterial imbalance. Most agreed that it was likely a combination of food sensitivities. The first idea that we decided to try was to make sure that I had absolutely no dairy in my diet at all. I was given a list of many foods where dairy can be hidden, and I worked on eliminating those.

Quinn's rash improved, and the diaper rash became less severe once I was very strict on avoiding dairy, which is incredibly hard when you love it! By now, Quinn was two months old and still having severe crying spells, watery and mucousy diarrhea, lots of gas and intestinal distress, and lots of forceful spit-up. He still had a rash and eczema all over his body. His doctor agreed that we needed to explore other foods to eliminate.

I began reading more and talking more with the ladies on my forum. I kept a log of everything I ate over the course of a week and discussed that log with the ladies on the forum. From that, they were able to point out some ideas. When Quinn was three months old, I removed caffeine and my vitamin supplements from my diet. Within a week, Quinn's bowel movements had become less watery, and his gas seemed less severe. He still had lots of mucus. The other symptoms were *still* unchanged.

During this time, my husband, a web programmer and statistician, decided he was going to figure this problem out. He coded a simple web app for me to record every single bite that I put in my mouth, and saved that information in a spreadsheet (unfortunately, this web app is still only source code. He has not had time to turn it into a real app.). I broke down every meal and snack into the major ingredients, eliminated several of the top allergenic foods, and plugged in. We knew this problem could be solved using this app. We just didn't know how long it would take.

When Quinn was four months old, I was desperately searching online using all sorts of combinations of words related to "fussy baby forceful spit ups," when I stumbled across a short response to a forum post buried somewhere on the web. I had an epiphany: what if chocolate is a problem? I started Googling like crazy and discovered that some people are sensitive to the mild stimulant in chocolate, theobromine. I also discovered that theobromine was in decaf tea, decaf coffee, acai berry, and several other foods. Since it was related to caffeine, sometimes people who are sensitive to theobromine are also sensitive to caffeine. I knew I had found the answer and promptly eliminated chocolate.

Within days, Quinn's crying spells reduced in severity, his gas almost completely disappeared, and his spitting up was greatly reduced. I was greatly encouraged, though I must admit that giving up chocolate was extremely difficult. I hadn't realized how much I depended upon it to get through my days. But through it all, I reminded myself that my baby wasn't wailing in pain for hours every day, and we were no longer going through five outfits and 10 spit-up cloths a day! We had found the food that really hurt him!

Finally, after a month of keeping very detailed food logs, my husband ran a statistical analysis on it. He confirmed that chocolate was closely correlated with severe distress in the baby, as well as my vitamins (which we had tried adding back into my diet) and, to our surprise, tomatoes. Eliminating tomatoes eliminated Quinn's eczema, and the remaining rash, remaining gas, diarrhea, and spit up. He was four and a half months old when he finally had clear skin, normal diapers, little to no spit-up, and the typical amount of gas.

It definitely took a village to figure that combination of food sensitivities out. Without the help of my online friends, Google, my husband, and the support of Quinn's doctor, we never would have worked it all out. I am very thankful for the resources we have available to us these days that allow us to make our lives better and solve so many problems that would have been dismissed as "just colic," or "just the way the baby is." I have continued to depend upon my online forum to help me figure out new food ideas, since most of the favorites on our menu included tomatoes and dairy.

Quinn is now a very active toddler who loves both nursing and solid food. We have slowly been testing the foods that he is sensitive to over the past couple months. He still cannot eat much tomato or chocolate, though I can have reasonable amounts of both. He gets a stomach ache from dairy, so I think that one's out for the long-run. I have found that since eliminating caffeine from my diet for a year, I now react to it rather badly, so I have chosen not to consume it often. I can take a few vitamin supplements, but if I take a multivitamin, Quinn still seems to have intestinal problems from it. Overall, I'm quite happy with how Quinn has outgrown the sensitivities so far, and am thrilled with every little bit of progress we make.

Chantal's Story

Breastfeeding has been a part of my whole life. I'm the oldest of seven children, all of whom were breastfeed, most past two years old. In addition, all of my mom's friends were breastfeeding mothers; most of them had large families, with five or more children, and never seemed to have any problems breastfeeding. In short, growing up, I was exposed to many boobies and lots of babies!

When I became pregnant, I thought breastfeeding would be no big deal after watching my mom effortlessly nurse my six younger siblings. A few weeks before my first son was to be born, a very nice woman from our church loaned me two books on breastfeeding. In the pages of those books, I learned the truth: breastfeeding is not always easy, nor is it always a natural instinct between mother and baby. I worried a bit, but again I wasn't starting from scratch. I had my mom, right? Somehow, it didn't occur to me that since being transferred to Hawaii for my husband's job in the military, I was now 4,000 miles away from her.

My first son, James, was born at home, and we didn't have too much trouble at first. We had some latch issues due to my inverted nipples, but my midwife offered support, and we seemed to be home free. When he was a week-and-half old, my son started crying; not a nice, gentle cry that could be soothed and helped—rather, a cry that lasted all day, and sometimes at night. I was dumbfounded on what to do to help him. As the weeks went by slowly I got more information. After chatting with my cousin on Facebook, she told me that she had to eliminate dairy products from her diet when she was nursing one of her children. My midwife also suggested it might be something I was eating. At my mother's suggestion, I Googled for help, and I came across a website that gave detailed instructions on how to eliminate dairy from your diet. Ten long days later, my son stopped the painful crying. Oh believe me, he still cried, but not that painful, sad crying he did before. Before I gave up dairy, he couldn't be soothed with breastfeeding, only eating as much as he could handle and then quitting. Slowly he started eating more at each meal. Eliminating dairy was totally worth it. I was dairy-free for five months, and partially dairy free for another six months. Once we figured out the problem, we enjoyed a nursing relationship that lasted 15 months.

Nineteen months after my first son was born, my second son joined the world. This time, I thought I'd have no problems. I was certain that he'd be okay and I wouldn't have to give up any food this time around. I mean, come on, my mom nursed seven kids and never gave up anything! After a wonderful home birth, Gideon and I had an easy start to our nursing relationship. It took my body about a week to get in the routine, and I had a little nipple pain, but it truly wasn't that bad. When he was a month old, I started having pain again. "I'll just wait it out," I thought, "it's probably from nursing too often at night or something." After about a week, it grew worse and worse until one of my nipples became cracked in five different places, and every time Gideon latched on, those cracks reopened. My skin was bright red on both breasts, which I thought was weird but just kept with it, until I finally I broke down because the pain was just too great. I told my husband I was ready to quit, I told my mom I was ready to quit, and that I had enough. I would sit crying holding my poor son (also crying) while I got up the nerve to latch him on. "Okay sweetie! Ready?? Mommy isn't ready. Okay, ready? One, two, three! OOOOWWWWWWW." For some reason, yelling out loud really helped me, although it was greatly disturbing to my little tyke.

Through my tears, my mom told me that it was not normal to have this pain, and I needed to perhaps do a little research to find the cause. "Maybe something's wrong," she said. "Have you searched online? Maybe you have thrush." So I started Googling my symptoms and thrush kept coming up as a possibility. At this point, I decided we needed to see a lactation consultant. Off we went—to the local hospital to seek professional advice. My mom was right! We were suffering from thrush. Getting through the bout of thrush was not easy, but we finally won our battle after two months! I found success with the home remedies that so many moms shared on their blogs and other breastfeeding resource sites. I truly couldn't have done it without them.

Thrush wasn't the only hurdle we had, though. Gideon also started crying nightly, for four to five hours, and was doing similar things that I had seen in his older brother: pulling his legs up, lots of gas, and a very distressed look on his face. I started with what I knew, and I gave up dairy. After three weeks, there was no change. I was so discouraged. I remembered all the research I did with James, and sadly, the next food to give up is wheat. I didn't want to do that at all. "It's not fair," I whined to my mom. "I hate breastfeeding." But guess what? I gave up wheat, and it made the biggest difference! All the crying stopped, and I had a happy baby again.

The online breastfeeding support I have gotten has been invaluable. I was clueless on how to eliminate all these foods from my diet. The blogs and websites other moms have taken time to write and organize are such great sources of information. Gideon is now nine months old and we love breastfeeding! Thanks to the advice I found online we are finally enjoying our nursing relationship!

Chapter 7

Exclusive Pumpers

Ask any mother who exclusively pumps her breast milk, and she will tell you that finding support to breastfeed in this capacity is hard! When I put out the call to mothers for this book, one of the first questions I received was: "I exclusively pump, does that count? Because to some, pumping and bottle-feeding isn't considered breast-feeding." I immediately answered, "Yes, of course you are considered a breastfeeding mom!"

For those mothers who do exclusively pump, it is hard to find support, and often they find their biggest cheerleaders online! Whether they pump exclusively because it is by choice, because of physiological reasons, or perhaps because they just didn't get off to the best start in the immediate postpartum period (a crucial window that can determine breastfeeding success) we should recognize that these mothers are extremely dedicated and literally work for every drop of milk they produce.

We often hear nursing mothers say they choose to breastfeed because they are lazy. There is nothing to prepare or wash as with bottle feeding, no trips to the store to buy formula and supplies, nothing to pack in a diaper bag before running errands. I argue that no matter how she feeds her baby, no mother is lazy, but there is certainly more work involved for breastfeeding mothers who exclusively pump. In addition to pumping milk, they have to wash and sterilize feeding supplies; prepare, label, and store their milk; all of this while keeping up with their babies' needs.

The logistics can be tricky if you add a pumping schedule to the time it takes to feed the baby, and this cycle can leave mothers exhausted. I had a friend who called me in tears in the early days of her breastfeeding relationship with her youngest child. Breastfeeding wasn't going as well as she hoped. She was pumping and supplementing what seemed around the clock and she felt a bit trapped, like she didn't have time to even run a quick errand before it was time to pump or feed her baby. She eventually was able to find a good rhythm, but in the midst of pumping, she needed support. The experience was overwhelming for her.

Other mothers are fortunate enough to create a pumping routine that works well for them and doesn't seem to dominate their schedules. I know another mother who had a preemie, born at 28 weeks, and she started pumping immediately after his birth. He was in a NICU that encouraged mothers to breastfeed, and she was fortunate enough, despite the stresses of having a baby in the hospital, to have a strong supply. She could easily pump more than enough to meet his needs. Because her baby was so little when he was born she didn't feed him at her breast, and upon bringing him home after a six-week stay in the hospital, she continued to pump and bottle feed.

She didn't always love pumping, and I think some days she dreaded it, but she found a way to make it work. She was able to get her body on a schedule that allowed her to pump four times a day, all while continuing to produce more-than-enough milk for her baby. Actually, she had a freezer full of milk and she ended up donating 2,500 ounces! She eventually was able to retire her pump at around eight months when her son spontaneously decided to latch on and feed from the breast. I share these two stories because they are two different mothers, with two different experiences—but both needed support. What works for one may not for another, but in the community that can be found online, the support needed to help a mother get through today's pumping schedule is priceless. It's important for these mothers to know that they aren't alone, and that there are other mothers to whom they can relate.

Rachel's Story

I am a 29-year-old mother of two amazing little boys. My oldest son, Sam, is four years old, and my youngest, Eli, is five months old. I am currently exclusively pumping breastmilk for Eli, and did the same thing for Sam when he was a baby.

I did not have any exposure to breastfeeding before I became a mom. I was the youngest child in my family, so I never saw a sibling being breastfed. I did hear stories growing up about how I breastfed until I was around age two, and how hard it was for me to give it up. Other than that, it wasn't something that we ever discussed. I made the decision before I had Sam that I would "try" to breastfeed, but I also gave myself permission that if it didn't work out, I'd be perfectly okay with it. I looked at a few articles online that I found through Google searches, but I didn't prepare too much for breastfeeding before I gave birth.

I had a planned cesarean section with Sam because I had a crushed pelvic bone from an accident when I was 18 years old, and that meant that it wasn't safe to deliver vaginally. Immediately after he was born, he was whisked away to the NICU because he was having trouble breathing. Apparently, this is common among c-section babies, but I didn't realize that at the time, and as a first-time mom I was terrified. I had asked to breastfeed him as soon as possible, but because of his breathing issues I didn't get to see him until he was 14 hours old. He was in an incubator for the first 24 hours, which meant no breastfeeding. By the time he was allowed to feed, the nurses had already given him formula.

A lactation consultant came to see me, and she gave me a breast pump and some very brief instructions. I felt alone, scared, and had absolutely no idea what I was doing, with no connection to breastfeeding help other than that provided at the hospital. Luckily, Sam and I came home after four days and settled in. I tried to get him to breastfeed, but I was so emotionally fragile I couldn't handle it. I rented a pump and I was resigned to exclusively pumping. I Googled what I could, but found out that most people either breastfed with occasional pumping, or formula fed. I was an oddity. I had terrible postpartum depression with Sam, and the pumping really added to my stress. After about four months, I decided to stop and switch to formula exclusively.

I finally became pregnant with Eli, my second son, after multiple miscarriages and surgery to correct a uterine septum. I had been through so much to get pregnant, and had dreamed of this little guy. It was incredibly important to me to breastfeed him successfully. By

85

the time he was born, I was using social media (Facebook and Twitter) more often and I also had a smart phone. I spent numerous hours researching any question that popped in my head. I liked Facebook's various groups, but because I hadn't given birth yet, I wasn't entirely involved. I bought all the breastfeeding supplies I could find. I was so prepared this time! I even had a postpartum care plan in place, which I felt would help tremendously. I couldn't wait to feel that bond with my newest little guy!

I had my planned c-section for Eli at 39 weeks and a few days, and when I caught a glimpse of him over the curtain after he was delivered, I fell in love! The nurses took his APGAR score while I waited. Then a pediatrician came into the OR and told me that he was being taken to the special care unit for infants, as I gave birth at a different hospital this time and it did not have a NICU. He had meconium in his sac and wasn't breathing correctly. I wasn't as stressed this time because of what I had experienced with Sam, but after a few hours, a specialist came in and explained that Eli would have to be moved to a different hospital because his breathing wouldn't improve, and the doctors thought they might need to intubate him. They whisked my baby away in an ambulance, and I was crushed. I specifically asked for a breast pump at this hospital because I knew what I had to do this time. The nurse provided one for me, and I went online to check how often I should be pumping. Every two hours I pumped, and it wasn't until after about two and a half days at the hospital that a lactation consultant came to see me. She gave me a number to call if and when I could do some "real" breastfeeding.

I was released from the hospital after three and a half days, but Eli couldn't be released because while he was in the NICU, the doctors discovered a congenital heart defect, and had to consult a cardiologist. I went directly from the hospital I was in to the NICU at the other hospital, and finally got to hold my baby. The nurses had been feeding him the little bit of milk I could pump, but mostly formula. I tried to breastfeed him, but he wasn't getting much (we weighed him before and after I fed). After his release, I tried my hardest to get him to take to my breast, but he was taking about 50 minutes per meal, and I had a four-year-old to take care of. I finally switched to exclusively pumping for him about two weeks after he came home.

I received a great deal of helpful breastfeeding information online during this time from La Leche League and KellyMom. I tried some Facebook groups, but I felt more comfortable with the evidence-based information I could access on these sites. It seemed like there was more information this time compared to four years earlier when I had Sam, or maybe I just knew how to find it better.

I would say I used online support almost constantly. I had my phone out multiple times a day searching for answers, and trying to find people who had gone through similar situations. I can't begin to explain how reassuring it is to find others who have to pump exclusively (although we're still a smaller group). From questions on the best pump to use, to how long to store the milk, and how to do it, I've found all my answers online. When you have a newborn baby, it is so much easier to find answers online than to haul yourself into a doctor's or lactation consultant's office.

I engaged in online activity mostly for the first two to three months. After my milk had evened out and I had a good schedule going, I found out I no longer needed it. Once in awhile I'll still have a random question, but not too often. I would say the Internet was invaluable to my breastfeeding relationship. Although I still didn't fulfill my dream of just breastfeeding my child, it helped me feel less alone in only pumping. It also answered every single question that would pass through my mind, and it has helped me to continue pumping for this long—I'm hoping to reach my goal of a year! I probably would have given up by this point if I didn't have the knowledge I gained online. The reiteration that breast milk is so great for babies' systems and most importantly, that breastfeeding and/or pumping is a real commitment, carried me through those times when I was ready to quit.

Breastfeeding turned out differently than I would have ever imagined. I never in my wildest dreams would have believed you if you told me I'd hook myself up to a machine multiple times a day that looks like I'm a cow being milked! All the knowledge that I gained from online resources helped make it possible for me to give my baby what I believe is the best food for him.

Jillian's Story

My name is Jillian, and my story is a little different than most breastfeeding mamas, as I am among the ranks of exclusively pumping mamas! I don't seem to fit in with the breastfeeding mothers, and yet I don't fit in with the formula-feeders either. Breastfeeding moms felt that I just couldn't get breastfeeding down and was lazy, and looked down at me for feeding my baby her bottle, even though it is my own breastmilk. I went so far as buying only bottles made by breast pump companies to almost broadcast to the world, "This is my breastmilk." The formula-feeding moms thought I was so strange for not just throwing in the towel and switching to formula. I was totally alone in a world by myself. My doctors and family said it couldn't be done. I had little support and nowhere to turn. On a whim, I decided to search the Internet to see if it was even possible to exclusively pump. I couldn't believe how much support there was for me, the mama who was so all alone, now surrounded by loving moms who had all been in my shoes and longed to help others.

Prior to my daughter's birth, I had decided early on I would breastfeed. My grandmothers had not breastfed, but my mom had. It was also helpful that I had an aunt due within two weeks of my due date who had breastfed all of her children. I did have support on hand from the start, but even with all the information in the world, breastfeeding is just something you have to do to understand.

After 19 hours, a Pitocin drip, and an epidural, my daughter was born. We had latch issues from the very beginning and I was given a nipple shield to use, which was supposed to make breastfeeding easier for us both, or so I thought. She really wanted nothing to do with nursing and just slept, and we had to keep waking her up to nurse. Looking back, I regret the medicated birth I had as I really think that had something to do with her being so tired and her "lazy" latch. The staff in the hospital had me try to nurse her for 30 minutes on a side every two hours with the shield. Before long, my nipples were raw and bleeding.

The day we left, she was diagnosed with jaundice, and we were required to return for tests every day for almost a week. Meanwhile, her diaper output indicated that she was becoming dehydrated, and the pediatrician requested that after every feeding I supplement with formula. At her daily weigh-ins I mentioned to the doctor that I was having breastfeeding difficulty, and she just told me to keep trying— she offered no additional help.

By this time, my nipples were beyond hurt, and I swear I cried more than she did when it came time to feed. I decided I was going to pump. Once I started pumping, I realized I had very little milk. I went online and looked up information on nipple shields and found that they might have actually been lessening my supply because I wasn't being stimulated enough. Why hadn't anyone at the hospital given me more information on nipple shields? This is when the reality of my breastfeeding relationship started to settle in, and I was completely devastated.

When my daughter was about 14 weeks old, I decided I'd had it with taking bad advice from people who tried to help me, and struck out online to salvage my badly damaged supply. I decided "I'm going to pump milk for this baby!" When I searched online, I couldn't believe how many moms were exclusively pumping—and not for short periods of time—some had been doing it for years! My aunt, who also had a newborn baby, gave me the sweetest gift of her milk for my daughter until my supply was built back up. For that, I will forever be grateful.

Following the advice of so many mothers before me, I got all the tricks of the trade: a better pump, a hands-free pumping bra, and tons of bottles. I dabbled in fenugreek, and when that didn't work, I ordered Motilium (Domperidone) from another country as it is not available in the United States. I changed my lifestyle completely. I pumped around the clock every two to three hours, and power pumped once a day. My breastfeeding experience has been so much more difficult than I could have ever imagined. "They" are right—it does not come naturally; it takes a lot of dedication and work, and in my case, plenty of blood, sweat, and tears—literally. I just marvel at women who nurse exclusively. I'm just thankful for every tiny drop of breast milk I'm able to provide her.

The online support system I found was incredible, and there are some moms who I will never actually meet, who have changed my life so much. While exclusively pumping resources are a little harder to find, there are in fact many groups, even groups for family members looking to support their pumping mamas. Those sites and ladies were there for me every hour of the day, all sitting on their computers while they were busy pumping. We were a sweet sisterhood of breastfeeding outcasts. We shared our secrets to building a supply, which is incredibly difficult when using just a pump, as no pump can ever remove as much milk as a hungry baby can. We shared our ups and downs, and counted every day and every ounce we pumped. We celebrated our goals with one another, and even cried over our spilled milk together.

I used their support for months, and actually still hang around the boards pretty frequently to pass on the information that was passed to me. I've never met another mother in my situation, but if I ever do, I will point her right online to read as much information as she could. I would also say don't be afraid to say you are an EP mom. I found it's so much easier when you know there are so many people supporting you. I even started keeping a little blog to document my breastfeeding journey. It's not really meant for others to read, but more a personal journal. Every once in awhile, I spot a visitor, and wonder what search term they typed into Google to find my site.

I do have to admit exclusively pumping is not for the faint of heart, doing the work of a nursing mother and a formula mother combined: just try feeding your baby a bottle while double pumping, and you'll understand. When my husband and I decided it was best for our family for me to wean, no one understood my feeling of being a total failure of a mother except my girls online. Some had weaned, and some had thoughts of it. The lifestyle of every two to three hours for months hooked to a pump, followed by the effects of the prescription galactogogues that need to be used can wear even the strongest of mamas down.

Eventually I realized I needed more freedom. I needed my husband and marriage back, and selfishly, maybe, I needed myself back. I was stuck on the edge of being a martyr and a sane woman. I had to be reminded by my EP sisterhood that anyone who had been in my shoes had long quit by now. I do believe that breast milk was the best nutrition for my baby, but maybe the motto should really be "every drop of breast milk makes a difference."

Part of me feels bitter that my breastfeeding journey never went as planned, but I have accomplished so much more than I ever thought, too. I had over six months to mourn the loss of breastfeeding, and my girls online helped me through it all. In time, the wounds will heal and I'll find myself on this road again giving it all I have, as I am pregnant again. I'm more afraid of breastfeeding than I am of labor. I long for that closeness of breastfeeding, but I know right where to find support and friendship online if I ever need to EP again.

I shared the following post with my Facebook group, Exclusively Pumping Moms (www.facebook.com/ExclusivelyPumpingMoms), the day my breastfeeding journey ended. It was the hardest day of my life, and I was completely heartbroken, but that heartbreak was followed by peace and joy. I'm so glad that the ladies of my group were there for me through it all and to see the last little miracle of my EP career:

> My little Zoey woke up earlier than normal today. She drank her six ounces of formula, but was still feeling a little restless; irritated she still had four more hours of sleep left. I was also feeling a little uncomfortable in my chest. I could feel there was not a lot, but some, milk in there. Not wanting to have to unpack my pump and put it all back together, I thought, "well, it doesn't hurt to see if she will latch one last time." Thinking to myself I don't have any idea where the nipple shield is, I prayed that she would latch onto me. I picked up my little miss and placed her in the football hold on a pillow. Took a deep breath ... and she latched. For the first time, on me, perfectly. There was no pain and my nipple didn't come out like a chewed tube of lipstick. She nursed very quickly, much quicker than the pump and not as strong. My heart melted the minute I saw the little drips of the last of my milk dribble out of the side of her mouth.

We had made it, she finally learned. Those last little drops were worth every minute of my bitter fight to breastfeed. While the moment only lasted several minutes, I just felt a total peace over the whole situation. As my little girl nursed herself to sleep one last time in my arms, I was finally thankful for all I was able to provide for her. I cuddled up next to her and thanked God for every drop she received.

Jennifer's Story

My name is Jennifer. I am now 47 years old and a very proud mother of three sons and one baby girl. I first became a mother at the age of 19, in 1985. I was young and immature, and could barely even say the word "breast" out loud. Through a single-mothers support group, I met a woman who introduced me to La Leche League. I attended meetings regularly, which provided me a ton of support to nurse my first baby for one year! I finished my A.A. degree in nursing in 1988, and started my career as a Registered Nurse. I had my second son in 1992, and was fortunate enough to nurse him for two years with no problems. Because it was before the Internet, I again attended some La Leche League meetings and always used their book, *The Womanly Art of Breastfeeding*, for support. Breastfeeding was so natural that I kept nursing my second until he was two, but I didn't tell anyone that he wasn't weaned. I even surprised a friend, who was not too keen on breastfeeding, when I told her that for about a year I was breastfeeding my son right in front of her, and she had been none the wiser!

I continued my professional nursing career, eventually earning my Master's in 2006, the same year that I remarried, and in 2007 became pregnant with my third son at the age of 41. I couldn't wait to breastfeed again, as it had been such an awesome experience with my first two sons. I even ordered a beautiful print of a woman nursing her child from the 1800s to decorate his room. All of my prenatal tests came back normal, and my anatomy ultrasound was also normal, so there was no way I could have been prepared for the surprise that occurred when he was born.

Within minutes of Luke's birth, the nurse who was cleaning him up while he screamed, caught a peek inside his mouth and said, "I think he has a cleft palate." I had heard of this but had no idea what it really meant. My birthing plan was to nurse him immediately after he was born, and there was to be no sugar water, pacifiers, or bottles. I didn't want anything to sabotage my efforts to nurse my baby, but this changed everything. They paged the pediatrician on call, as it was 11 p.m., so no one was really around, and he said, "she can try to breastfeed." My plan was to get back to my room and try to nurse him. As soon as they admitted me to the mother/baby unit, they took one look at Luke having trouble with his own secretions, as the sinuses are connected to the mouth through the open palate, and put a sign on his little bed that said "spitting." I was told he was going to be kept in the nursery overnight and observed, and I was told to go to sleep and rest. I was sick with worry for my baby and distraught about not being able to nurse him right away.

Sometime the next morning, they brought him in. I eventually tried to nurse, and even though it had been more than 16 years, I still felt like I knew what to do. When we tried to breastfeed, he would start to latch on, and then immediately there was no suction, and therefore no nursing, because he could not latch and stay on my breast. They brought me a pump and I started pumping every three hours. I pumped colostrum in syringes, and we started trying to just squeeze that in his mouth. He did not know what to do with a syringe and tongue thrusting was an issue. The lactation consultant came to help us with a textbook and all kinds of equipment: nipple shields, syringes, tubing, and a bottle called a Habermann bottle for special feeding. The bottle was given to me, but no one really knew how it worked.

The textbook was to explain to me, an experienced nurse mind you, that it is impossible to nurse a baby with a cleft palate; because his palate, which included the muscles to suck, basically had a hole in it, creating a seal to facilitate breastfeeding was impossible. I was not willing to accept this; I was in denial, and I was so against formula and bottles that I was determined my son would not get a drop of formula. The nurses after each shift would ask me how long "I nursed." All I could think to myself was, "Hello, my baby can't nurse!" I was feeding milliliters of colostrum at a time, which was really all I was making anyway. Before long, we realized he was dehydrated and jaundiced, and ended up staying an extra day to be treated with bili lights.

When Luke came home, our plan was for me to use a nipple shield, put him on the breast and squeeze the breast milk through the syringe into tubing into his mouth so he knew where it was coming from. Of course he could not suck, so I pumped every three hours and attempted to nurse this starving child every two hours. Feeding him seemed to take forever; it took probably an hour to try to feed him through this apparatus. I think I slept maybe one hour for every six in between. It was absolutely insane!

I took him into the pediatrician the next day. He was jaundiced, dehydrated, and losing weight, and she sent me to the cleft palate clinic at Rady Children's Hospital. They saved my baby's life and mine. They again reiterated that I was not going to be able to nurse and they gave me a bottle designed for a cleft palate. I had brought breast milk with me. We put it in the bottle and squeezed, and the milk shot into his mouth. I continued trying to nurse a couple times a day, but with pumping every three hours, and 20 minutes spent feeding him so that he did not spend all his calories trying to eat, I ended up running out of time trying to nurse him. I put him against my bare breasts every time I fed him his bottle so he had exposure to my skin and could feel the closeness of nursing. I continued to offer him the breast in hopes that after he had surgery, I could teach him to nurse. When he was three months old, I tried to nurse him. I put my nipple in his mouth, he gagged, and I knew it was over. It was a sad day for me. I never could bring myself to hang the picture of the baby nursing I had bought for his nursery because it was too painful for me.

I was not going to give up, so I continued to pump. I initially rented a hospital-grade pump for about a month, and then I got my own double-electric pump. I searched the Internet for support, and I was able to connect with other moms through a Yahoo! group called "Exclusive Pumpers." We were all pumping because our babies could not nurse for medical reasons. These mothers were my life! Any question I had, they knew it all; every ounce of information from troubleshooting pump problems—the babies, calories, and timing—everything was there for me at my fingertips.

I went back to work when Luke was six months old, and I bought a car adaptor so that I could maintain my supply and keep pumping regularly. With my pumping bra, I learned how to pump while I drove, (talk about cell phones and texting, I was pumping and could change bottles if they filled while driving—I wouldn't recommend this). I also had battery pack, and could walk around while pumping!

I was determined my son would only receive breast milk for as long as possible, so my pumping was essential. I needed to maintain my supply by pumping as often as possible. This was a different, very stressful feeling compared to breastfeeding. My baby was dependent on my pumping. My life was pumping. If I left the house, I had to have my pump or breast milk so I could feed my baby. I had no other way to feed him. The nice thing is that my husband could feed him this wonderful milk, which allowed me time to pump.

I could not have done this without my husband, because he knew how important it was to me that Luke received my breast milk, and he fully supported me. I often sat in the back seat of the car while he drove and I pumped. To maintain my supply, I used fenugreek capsules and tea. I used every strategy to increase supply, including power pumping, where I essentially would pump every 15 minutes for an hour, and do that every time my supply dropped. I had a period where it just started dropping despite all my efforts. I had heard of the medication Reglan being used from my EP'ers group, so I asked my doctor to order it for me. I wasn't able to take it three times a day, as prescribed, because it made me very tired, but I did take it every night, and it was helpful. I continued to take it until I stopped pumping. Unfortunately, Luke had very slow weight gain despite all my pumping efforts. At one point, a nutritionist recommended that I add formula to his diet. He was close to a diagnosis of failure to thrive, and this was attributed to the calories he burned while trying to get milk. We eventually decided that he needed the formula, so we added the supplements.

Luke had full palate reconstruction at ten months of age. I was able to stay with him and pump through his hospital stay. Because I was pumping, the hospital provided me all my meals, and kept my milk refrigerated so my son could have it when able to take food by mouth. I felt so supported and admired for nursing this cleft-palate child. Nurses and doctors always commended me and said what a gift that was and how incredible it was to still be giving him breast-milk. I continued to pump for one year, my supply having greatly diminished after Luke's surgery, and I was gradually adding more and more formula—but Luke received breastmilk for one year and that was my goal.

In February of 2012, at the age of 46, I learned I was pregnant again. Surprised, anxious, and scared, I soon learned that I was carrying a healthy baby girl. She was born in September, perfect as can be, and I nursed her immediately after birth. She is an eager little nursling, and I am once again experiencing one of life's greatest gifts, breastfeeding and nurturing my child with my body as God meant for me to do.

I have been able to breastfeed all of my children successfully thus far, but if it had not been for the resources I found online when Luke was a baby, I would have probably not met my breastfeeding goal. Finally, I have the breastfeeding picture from the 1800s on the wall in my daughter's nursery, and it doesn't make me sad anymore.

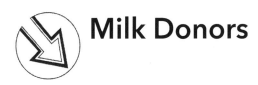 # Milk Donors

Breastmilk has sustained human life on this planet since the appearance of modern man. If we could travel back in time, I bet we would find examples of milk-sharing from very early on. Red deer, buffalo, bighorn sheep, and pigs all practice allosuckling—when female animals cross-nurse other animals' young—so the practice is not unheard of in the animal kingdom. Many scientific studies have tried to figure out why animals do it, and whether or not the practice is beneficial or detrimental. The results have been varied and no generalizations across species can be drawn. What matters for us, I suppose, is that we aren't the only mammals who see the value of, or need to share milk. When we realize that human milk is a precious commodity in great demand, sharing among mothers can be life-saving to babies in need. The use of donor milk in hospitals for babies in NICUs is increasing, as it is recognized as being the healthiest choice for preemies and medically fragile infants. Additionally, in hospitals where it is available, donor milk can be used to supplement newborn babies whose mothers are experiencing a delay in milk production.

Milk sharing can be a sensitive subject as some people are not comfortable with the idea of giving their baby another mother's milk. Our society definitely has some reservations with regard to sharing and donating breastmilk—it is seen as dirty or gross, when in reality is neither of those. Two recognized kinds of milk sharing are practiced: formal and informal. In the United States and Canada, formal milk sharing is when human milk is donated through non-profit milk banks, which are members of the Human Milk Banking Association of North America (HMBANA). HMBANA has standards to which all member banks must adhere, and milk collected through these banks is regulated and controlled. Just as blood donors go through an approval process and their blood donations are screened for pathogens, milk donors are screened before their donations are accepted and their milk is screened and pasteurized before being sent to hospitals. Milk banks and depots are emerging all over the country to meet the increased demand for human milk as education creates awareness for this valuable and precious commodity.

Informal milk sharing is when mothers donate their milk directly to friends, family, or others. Wet nursing is the oldest form of informal milk sharing, and while the practice can still be found it is rare, and the vast majority of breastmilk informally shared is done with a breast pump, and often frozen and stored immediately after it is collected. While informal milk sharing is a blessing for many, families who take milk informally must take necessary steps to ensure the milk they give their babies is safe, as it is possible to transmit illness through breastmilk. Are there risks one must weigh when using donor milk that does not come from a milk bank like HMBANA, which has a strict screening process and pasteurizes and tests milk before sending it to hospitals? Of course, but many parents believe the benefits of informal milk sharing outweigh the risks of using infant formula.

Human Milk 4 Human Babies and Eats on Feets are two of the largest and best-known global online milk-sharing networks that allow parents to connect with donors. The process is simple: you search by location, post your need, and wait for contact! These sites do suggest a protocol to follow when choosing a donor, but leave the individuals to work out the details of their arrangements on their own. Breastfeeding mothers are often very generous in taking the time to pump and store their extra milk, and often helping to transport it to the family in need. While the majority of donor milk recipients are forever grateful, the mothers who donate are thrilled to be able to share their milk and not have it go to waste! Our society is moving toward greater acceptance of donor milk, and hopefully in the years to come we will see milk banks as plentiful as blood banks, and even "Milk Mobiles" that can host donor milk drives! In the meantime, mothers will keep sharing and babies will keep receiving the wonderful gift of milk.

Chelsea's Story

I remember my mom brought my siblings and me to La Leche League meetings when my brother was a baby. He nursed until he self-weaned at around three years old. I remember my mom's breast pump and stacks of breastfeeding books and magazines in the living room on the side table, and I remember playing with the breast pump. Now my mom reminds me that I used to nurse my toy babies along with her. It's no surprise when I found out I was pregnant with my first, I knew I would breastfeed. Mom gave me all her books and magazines to read during the pregnancy, and I excitedly did as I waited for the birth of my first baby.

Finally, the time came and I gave birth to a precious little girl. We were overjoyed! I immediately put her to my breast, and she latched on without much difficulty. I was in heaven for about five minutes, then it all came to a crashing halt. The nurse ripped my little girl from my breast and put an oxygen mask over her because she was turning blue. She couldn't breathe. We later found out her breathing difficulty was because of a pneumothorax. She was sent to the NICU about two hours from the hospital where I was, and I didn't see her again until almost 24 hours later. We spent three days with her in the NICU, without any breastfeeding support, and every time I tried to breastfeed, I was discouraged because she wasn't supposed to leave the air tank for too long. We just had to settle for quick cuddles.

When we finally arrived home, I followed my instincts and tried nursing again. I felt that it was starting to go well. She was eager to nurse. We had one home visit from a nurse who told me I was starving my child and needed to stop, so I did. What type of mother would I be if I kept nursing and killed my own daughter because of my selfishness?

Three years later I became pregnant with our second child. This time I was educated and angry over how my daughter and I were treated. This time was going to be different. I found a Traditional Birth Attendant (TBA) and I attended La Leche League meetings during my pregnancy. I explained to everyone what happened with my first baby, and expressed my fears over it happening again. I did even more reading and Googling about breastfeeding than I did with my first because this time nothing was going to stop me. My son's birth was wonderful. He was born at home in our bathtub. He latched on within an hour after being born, and it looked like breastfeeding was actually going to happen for us. I couldn't be happier.

By day three, he was constantly fussing and on the breast 24/7. I knew something was wrong, I could just feel it in my gut. He hadn't been weighed again since birth, so I had no clue if he was gaining or not. I was on the phone crying to my mom and she suggested a few things to try, like different nursing positions. I called the La Leche League hotline and received tips over the phone from a lovely lady. She also sent me a few links to different sites to help me out. I called my TBA for more suggestions and support. She told me to start pumping in an attempt to increase my supply. She also suggested taking fenugreek with blessed thistle. If that didn't help, we would then try Domperidone.

I pumped constantly. While he was nursing, I would pump the other breast. When he wasn't nursing, I was pumping. I would take a bath and bring the hand pump with me. I would wake up with my son and pump a few times throughout the night. I was exhausted and so stressed out because I never saw any change, but I was determined to make it happen.

A week later, things were not getting better. He was screaming because he was so hungry, and had lost an unhealthy amount of weight. He was dehydrated and it broke my heart. We got out the formula sample the company sent us and gave him something to eat. At first, I had my husband use a little eye-dropper and drop formula onto my breast close to his mouth. That way he was still on the breast, but getting something more. Our TBA suggested using a Supplemental Nursing System (SNS). Seeing my son nurse happily on the breast with an SNS made me cry. This was not the way it was supposed to happen; I studied and tried so hard to get it right this time around. I hated to see the formula leave the bottle and go into my baby boy's tummy. It was heart-wrenching to watch, and made me feel like a failure as a mother. There was nothing anyone could do to cheer me up. I was slowly swirling into a pit of depression again.

I started to join different groups and pages on Facebook. I was looking for support, tips, a magical supply-increasing cure to my breastfeeding problems; I was desperate. First, I joined a page called Peaceful Parenting, and one day they did a shout out to groups. One group was called Informed Choice: Birth and Beyond/HM4HB. There, I met a great group of women who tried to help me out, giving me tips. They really cheered me up and gave me hope. There was one woman who I met who had the same issues I was having. She finally increased her supply and was able to get rid of the SNS. In the end, she actually ended up being able to donate extra milk she had. Her story renewed my strength and helped to push me forward and to keep trying.

A few weeks later, we were still using the SNS. Nothing had changed. With all my hard work, nothing had changed. Our TBA suggested getting donor milk from another mom. At first I thought, "That is so gross–what about diseases and bacteria?" I nodded and smiled, and said we would think about it. Really though, I had no interest. Formula was good enough for my daughter. It will just have to be fine for my son too, especially since its usage would only be temporary.

I pushed the thought of donor milk to the back of my mind, and didn't think about it again until the creator of the group Informed Choice: Birth and Beyond, Emma Kwasnica, started to talk about Human Milk 4 Human Babies, posting articles and blogs about donated human milk. It made me very curious because we had just heard about donated milk from our TBA. I looked into it, and was slammed with all this information. Emma then went on to establish a worldwide community to help parents in need get donor milk. When I saw there was a group for my province, I joined the community.

By this time, my son was about two months old. He had been using the SNS with formula for the last month and a half, and we knew that this was going to be for the long run now. We weighed the risks between formula and breastmilk, and did a great deal of research. My husband and I finally made the decision to ask for milk donations from the group Human Milk 4 Human Babies. I was so nervous to ask for milk, and was not sure what was going to happen, but I had to try because in my gut I felt it was the best decision for us.

My first request was met with many offers. It was wonderfully overwhelming. They offered advice and tips. A few women even private messaged me to see how they could help. I can't remember the exact amount of women willing to donate their milk to my son, but we received at least seven to ten offers. We contacted each one, and thus started our journey into receiving donated milk. I continued to pump like a mad woman, taking galactagogues,

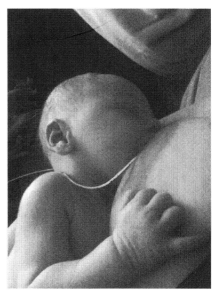

Chelsea's second son, five days old, nursing with the SNS. —*Photo credit: Chelsea Casson*

and I don't think I have ever eaten so much oatmeal with brewer's yeast in my life—all to get my supply to increase. I did this until my son was a year old.

Our family was blessed again, and we had a third child, a little boy. When he was born, I had so much more knowledge on how to increase supply, and I really felt like I was ready. I bought a new pump, stocked up on herbs to help with supply during pregnancy, and planned our second homebirth. Immediately after birth, he initiated breastfeeding, and I continued to nurse my toddler. I started pumping soon after to help bring in my milk, and by day three all the signs that I was not making milk happened again. By day four, our newborn had lost more than a pound, so we had to start supplementing again. This time I knew how to use an SNS, and had a couple moms ready to donate in the event we needed it again.

I wanted to know why I was unable to produce milk, so I went to a lactation consultant who told me that I am one of the rare moms who have insufficient glandular tissue (IGT). She said there was nothing I could do. I was—and am—devastated. I went online and found a website dedicated to moms with IGT. There, I found another Facebook page for IGT and chronic-low-milk-supply moms. This became my village; it's where I feel I belong. These women understand what I am going through and are supporting me through this mourning process. They get where I am coming from, the hardships and the guilt. It's really nice to finally fit in somewhere, where the norm is low supply and supplementing. If it wasn't for this group, I would have been lost alone in a world where people don't understand (including my care providers). It is a scary and depressing place to be.

On my journey as a breastfeeding mom, I have found so much support online. I am no stranger to online support, as my husband is in the military. I have found many of groups on Facebook and Twitter with women whose husbands or partners are also serving in the Canadian military. Finding online groups for breastfeeding and parenting support came pretty easily. If it were not for online support I am sure I wouldn't still be breastfeeding. I would have given up without the women online cheering me on. I feel as though online support is almost as crucial in my life as real-life support, and I am so grateful that it exists. Because of the support I received online, I have now started to pursue a career in lactation education and as a childbirth educator. I want to impart the knowledge these ladies gave to me, and I want to support other women the way my friends online have supported me.

Hillary's Story

My memories of my younger siblings do not involve them being breastfed. I remember formula being mixed and nipples being sterilized–a very scientific process–but I have no memory of seeing them on my mother's breast, which is sad, really, because my mom fought long and hard for all of her babies, and only four of us survived and lived. It seems almost disrespectful to remember breastfeeding as the battle she lost.

My pregnancy was a surprise. I was working a high-stress job, and becoming pregnant meant selling our too-small condo and moving to a new city. My pregnancy was filled with to-do lists, moving boxes, and navigating the minefield my job became once my pregnant status was disclosed. The extent of my preparation–for both childbirth and breastfeeding–was a weekend course run by a local midwife. She did an excellent job covering childbirth, but time constraints meant that the breastfeeding portion of the course was cut short. She whipped out a crocheted breast at the end of day two and held a doll up to the nipple so we could observe a perfect latch. Late in my pregnancy, a doctor (the practice I went to had eight doctors on rotation) asked if I was planning to breastfeed. I replied that I was planning to try. That was it, there was no further discussion about it.

I went into labor naturally five days after my due date. I had an uncomplicated labor, and my son was born without the aid of an epidural about seven hours after I was admitted to the hospital. My labor-and-delivery nurse brought him to my breast within minutes of his birth, and he latched on immediately. I stayed in the hospital for a little over a day, and he spent the majority of that time latched onto my breast. The doctors and nurses all told me I was doing such a fantastic job because he was so content to suckle. I didn't question the intense pain I felt. I thought that it was normal and would abate once my body adapted.

My son's intense drive to suck did not let up when we were released from the hospital. I suffered at home for two days before my husband begged me to get help. My nipples were cracked and raw. My toes would curl with pain, and I would choke back sobs when my son latched onto me. Tears streamed down my face as I fed my son for what felt like the thousandth time. On the third day of my son's life, my husband walked me over to the public health office (conveniently located a block away from our home), and I mournfully showed the nurse my mangled nipples. She showed me how to improve my son's latch, and how to hold him so that he wasn't pulling down on my nipples. She weighed him and noted that he had already gotten back up to–and passed–his birth weight, which was something positive for me to focus on. I left feeling much more optimistic about breastfeed-ing. The only problem was that even though our latch had been fixed, I was still faced with having to nurse my son with my damaged and extremely painful nipples.

I am a blogger, and Twitter and Facebook are part of my daily life. I have a wide network of friends whom I've never met. When I faced my first breastfeeding challenges, Twitter was the first place I turned to. None of my local girlfriends have kids, so I turned to my virtual girlfriends for support. Twitter got me through the first few weeks of breastfeeding. The first night after my appointment with the nurse, when I couldn't tell if her corrections were actually helping because my injured nipples were still so painful, a Twitter friend told me I could quit "tomorrow." All I had to do was get through the night and I could quit tomorrow. Everything seemed better in the light of day, and it would get me through to another night. That carried me through the first few weeks while my nipples slowly healed. Once my breasts healed and nursing was no longer excruciatingly painful, my Twitter friends became more of a support group than a crisis line. We used the hashtag "zombiemoms," and chatted during late-night feedings. Talking to other nursing mamas carried me through months of fractured sleep.

I had an oversupply of milk. My son flat-out refused to take a bottle, so I tried not to pump as I didn't want to increase my supply even more. I often had to pump to relieve the pressure. I ended up with a freezer full of milk for which I had no use. My son was about five months old when I was finally being treated for the postpartum depression and anxiety I had silently suffered from since days after he was born, and happened to discover that I lived near a human milk bank. I contacted them and went through the screening process. Donating my extra breast milk—and knowing that I was helping other babies–healed me in a way that therapy, counseling, yoga, and Ativan couldn't. I wouldn't have been able to be a breast milk donor if I had quit breastfeeding in the early days when I was struggling so hard.

I went back to work full-time when my son was six months old. I pumped in the (70s style, complete with orange fixtures) bathroom every day, multiple times a day. I talked to other mamas on Twitter while I pumped, I posted pictures of my pumped milk, and I cheered on other women who were doing the same. Twitter provided me a cheering squad.

I left my high-stress job when my son turned a year old to become a work-at-home mom. He is 17 months old now and we are still breastfeeding. I honestly believe that we're where we are today because of the support I received online. My partner, my family, my friends–they are all great sources of strength and support for me, but they can't always be there in the moment. Twitter provided that instant encouragement. At any given time, I could tweet about nipple blisters or spilling five ounces of freshly expressed milk, or my jerk boss who was complaining about how much time I wasted pumping, and I would have an instant interaction with someone who gave me a little boost to keep going. So much of the first year of breastfeeding–for me–was just making it through to the next feeding.

My advice to pregnant women who are considering breastfeeding is to prepare yourself before you give birth. Make the connections online before you need them. I was lucky enough to already use Twitter, so I had friends and followers. I already had my "team," even though I didn't know it at the time. Make the connections, find the support, and figure out where you can go online if you do end up needing help–because chances are you will need help. Breastfeeding is a challenge, but it is one of the most rewarding things I've done with my life. I am so grateful for the support I found online. I wouldn't be where I am now without it.

Chapter 9

Too Little, Too Much: IGT and BFAR

Breasts permeate our culture, and sadly most often not in a way that promotes breastfeeding. From a very early age, we are exposed to countless examples of ideal breasts that appear big, round, and firm. Before our breasts even start to develop, we have ideas of how they are supposed to look. Then puberty strikes, our bodies change, and without any input from us, we develop the breasts we were destined have by genetics. They never do quite look like the ones we saw growing up—and how could they? The breasts plastered in advertisements, which we can't ever get away from, aren't even real—they are man-made.

Sadly, we don't figure out until much later in life that breasts are more than just eye candy, they are intended to provide us pleasure during sexual encounters, and of course, nature intended them as a life-source for our babies. Between the emergence of our breasts and pregnancy and breastfeeding, we often spend time disliking our breasts. Some women are bothered by their breasts because they are too big and cause them physical discomfort. Other women just want even breasts, as one may tend to be a little larger than its counterpart. Of course, countless women think their breasts are too small and not full enough. Our breasts can't win: they are either the wrong size, not perky enough, the nipples are too big or small, the wrong color, etc. The bottom line is that we often take our breasts for granted, and spend time cursing them for not growing into the perfect pair, never even thinking that one day we are going to need them—that our babies are going to need them.

Statistics for 2011 show that in the United States there were more than 590,000 cosmetic and reconstructive surgical procedures involving women's breasts (American Society of Plastic Surgeons, 2012). Each year this number rises; even in times of economic hardship, we as a society still take time to surgically alter our breasts. It is important to note that not all women are receiving surgery to make their breasts larger. Tens of thousands seek surgery for reasons other than vanity. For example, many women undergo breast-reduction surgery because they suffer with pain related to heavy breasts. Other women just want their breasts to appear symmetric. And of course there are women who have reconstructive surgery due to illness, such as breast cancer.

While there is no definitive statistic, the best estimate among lactation support professionals presumes that about five percent of women can't breastfeed due to reasons related to maternal physiology. If we are looking at the mother and her body, it could be due to breast surgery (augmentation or reduction mammoplasty), or a condition known as hypoplasia or Insufficient Glandular Tissue (IGT), which results in lactation failure. Sadly, women who suffer from IGT often don't know they have it until they try breastfeeding and realize early on that they aren't producing enough milk.

> *The Breastfeeding Answer Book* cites a 1999 estimate that 1 in 1,000 mothers experience primary lactation failure, which can be due to hypoplasia or other causes. However, with an increasing number of mothers becoming pregnant and delivering healthy babies who previously could not, thanks to assisted fertility and hormonal support, more cases of hypoplasia are being encountered. This increase has occurred because many conditions that underlie problems achieving and sustaining a pregnancy coexist with insufficient breast development. Some of these red-flag conditions may give a mother or her health care providers clues to a future lactation failure if they are aware of them early in pregnancy." (Cassar-Uhl, 2009)

As we all know, pregnancy comes with major changes to our bodies and our minds; being caught off guard and facing the reality of not making enough milk to support a growing baby during this fragile time can be extremely difficult. Thank you Naomi, Amanda, and Kelly for sharing your stories so poignantly, sharing what worked for you to help you meet your breastfeeding goals, and helping us realize that there is support for those faced with possible lactation failure.

Naomi's Story

My breastfeeding story probably starts at puberty. Well, it could even start way back when I was just a speck in my mother's womb, as she watched the crop dusters spray the tomato plantations in the town she lived, with its semi-agricultural setting, alongside the backdrop of a busy coke (coal) works and shipping port. I mention this because although my mother had no problems breastfeeding me (her fourth child) for 12 months, there is increasing literature to suggest that dioxins, and exposure to pollution in fetal development, could play a part in affecting how this little speck goes on to breastfeed.

Everything seemed to be ticking away and ripening during adolescence, apart from one frustrating issue. Where were these breasts that all my friends were sprouting? I would get out my mother's sewing measuring tape, check my stats against my clothing labels with their size guide. You know the one I'm talking about in many children's clothes (thank heavens they don't have them for grown ups). Hips and waist, all checked out, but the only bust measurement I could come up with was, well, busted, surely? Nowhere near the stated size!

To cut a long story short, things eventually started to develop in my late teens, albeit only on my right side. I was really uneven, and both of my areolas were strange and puffy, kind of like googly eyes. If I bought a bra, I couldn't have filled an AA cup on the left. The right was just shy of a B cup. We muddled along stuffing foam inserts in that recalcitrant side, but it really affected my self-confidence. My mother—probably feeling guilty that she had somehow "caused" this—paid for me to have breast implants when I was 20 years old. Because I was diagnosed by the plastic surgeon with "tuberous or hypoplastic breast deformity" (or Insufficient Glandular Tissue as it's called in breastfeeding circles), some of the cost was covered by health insurance. This was to be the last I thought about them, or that diagnosis really, until I was pregnant in my late 20s.

I work as a clinical nurse in a busy tertiary hospital NICU. I see breasts everywhere, help mothers deal with expressing or breastfeeding most days. I thought I knew it all! Only once in my time as a nurse did I ever see a pair that looked like mine, when I took an electrocardiogram on an older woman in emergency early in my nursing career. Considering the number of breasts I see each day, I guess that means I was pretty rare! Most times, it seemed the consensus on the NICU floor was that if a mother wasn't bringing enough milk in to feed the baby, she probably wasn't "doing enough." I know better now.

I started to get worried when I was pregnant about how it would go with feeding after not only having surgery to my breasts, but knowing how little tissue was there to begin with. My obstetrician didn't really care (or for that matter, look at them during antenatal visits when I told her about my breast condition). I quietly asked around my work. The answer seemed to be, "of course, even small breasted women can feed!" usually accompanied by a glance to my (ample) chest—I certainly didn't look small. Because I was working on writing policies at the time, I was pretty clued up on doing scholarly

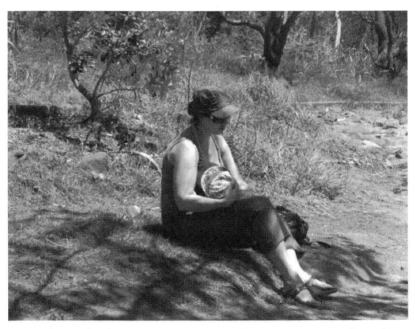

Naomi breastfeeding her oldest son, Lachlan, on a nature walk. —*Photo credit: Naomi Drew*

literature searches, and I ran some journal article searches on breast hypoplasia. I couldn't find much that wasn't plastic-surgery literature, which made no mention of breastfeeding, of course!

I eventually had my first baby, Lachlan, by emergency c-section, after he became distressed after a long, induced labor. Things went pretty pear-shaped with feeding. He wasn't gaining back the large amount of weight he lost in hospital, was unsettled, and nappy outputs were down, along with "brick dust" or urates in his nappy on day seven. I was probably in some form of denial about how well he was feeding to not pick up on the issues until he was ten days old, given my breastfeeding knowledge from work. My nipples were shredded for the first month until he could have a tongue-tie fixed. Oh how I cried when we bought that first tin of formula, and I felt like such a failure and so alone. I couldn't talk to my friends. They all seemed to feed so effortlessly, often for two years.

I sought help from an IBCLC at my hospital clinic when he was about two weeks old, who agreed my lack of glandular tissue from my tuberous breasts meant I had trouble making enough milk. But with medication to boost my prolactin levels (Domperidone), and a whole lot of pumping, I managed to feed my son. Sometimes exclusively, sometimes with formula top ups via bottle, for around eight months, until I fell pregnant with my second son. But man, was it tiring. The whole "nurse, top up, express, try to get him to sleep, and then repeat, ad infinitum" merry-go-round was pretty exhausting. I never could feed off the left side; he fussed and cried on it. I never had let downs or expressed more than 5mL of milk off it, but could manage to limp along okay on my right. Eventually he stopped wanting to nurse on the left, and I just nursed on the right. For some reason, Lachlan was particularly sensitive to hormonal changes in my milk, and flat out refused to nurse once I became pregnant.

I wasn't diagnosed with perinatal mood disorders (PMD), but was pretty down on myself for a while for how things played out. I couldn't do his baby book for a long time, as seeing those pictures of him those first couple of weeks, with a drawn little mouth and frown, how hungry he must have been, and I just couldn't hear him screaming it to me. I did some searching on my feelings and stumbled

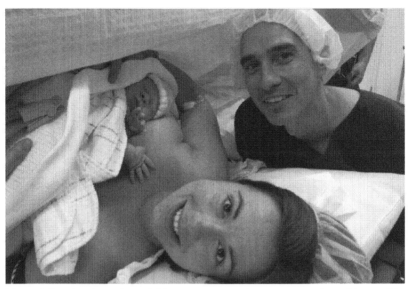

Naomi, her husband, and Eli, their second son, practicing skin to skin after her c-section. —*Photo credit: Naomi Drew*

across a blog by Dr. Alison Stuebe on the Academy of Breastfeeding Medicine page. She wrote something really powerful, "When Lactation Doesn't Work," which just made me feel so understood, and that there were health professionals out there who didn't think I wasn't trying hard enough to make milk. Through this subscription, I saw the recommendation to join a Facebook group for mothers with IGT later when my second son was five months old. I wish I had known about the support group for mothers with IGT with my first baby.

Things were going to be different with my second breastfeeding journey. I was adamant. I had my favorite book, *The Breastfeeding Mother's Guide to Making More Milk*, by Diana West and Lisa Marasco, and a plan to ensure some obstacles to maximizing my milk supply would be minimized. And so, Eli was born. I had a planned caesarean, but was able to have skin to skin for close to half an hour while they stitched me up. I had unrestricted breastfeeding and minimal visitors. If he blinked, he was put on the boob! I started Domperdione early on day three (much to the grumbles of my obstetrician who didn't think it did anything that early). I made the pediatrician check for tongue-tie, who cleared him of it, saying "what a great suck he has, look how he can stick his tongue out!"

But nursing hurt. It really hurt, and to boot I had these weird white blisters, and a flattened nipple no matter how I held him. I had "textbook positioning" according to the IBCLCs who visited me in hospital. But he would stumble and choke during feeds, and swallow so much air I could feel it through his back as he nursed. I searched Google to find answers as to why this was happening, and came to the conclusion that it could be over-active milk ejection reflex (OAMER). The KellyMom website had a great article on it, and I thought the flattening was due to him clamping down to slow the flow, which had also been suggested to me from the baby nurse at my local chemist. I've often found KellyMom to be my first port of call for breastfeeding-related issues; even better now that she has an article on IGT!

I just didn't think things were right, and saw another IBCLC at four months. Without putting her finger in his mouth, she told me he didn't look tongue tied, but said he had an upper lip tie. I saw it mentioned on my IGT Facebook group that lip ties are often associated with hidden posterior (submucosal) tongue-ties. Things started whirring in my mind. I did more searches. IBCLC Catherine Watson Genna's website (www.cwgenna.com) was invaluable in teaching me how to check for a posterior tongue-tie, and I became very suspicious he had one. My husband thought I was making mountains out of molehills and I shouldn't have been diagnosing stuff off the net. I asked our dentist what to do about the lip tie, one of the reasons I felt he couldn't get a great latch, and he didn't think they treated it until adult teeth came through. After many fruitless phone calls to different providers, I eventually got an appointment with the doctor who did a scissor frenotomy on my eldest son's tongue tie, just to see if he would do the lip tie and check his tongue.

I say this a lot, being a mother of course, but heck, I was right! He did have a posterior tongue-tie. We had it and his lip tie clipped, and although there wasn't the 100% relief I felt with my eldest son, things were better. Sadly, five months of scary choking while nursing took its toll on my little Eli, who would throw a nursing strike at the drop of a bra clip, and made my supply all the more fragile and prone to dips until I could woo him back. I found online other ways to help my supply through herbal tinctures instead of choking down fenugreek, alfalfa, and blessed thistle capsules, and I weaned off Domperidone around six months. I even was able to buy these herbs much cheaper than in-store by searching around online. Many days I had to exclusively pump; others, he would give me brief respite and be okay with nursing. It was getting me down that I could just make enough milk, but he hated nursing. I held on to the hope that I gained from my friends on the Internet that I should never "quit" on a bad day, and that things could improve. How right they were! I had support and friendship from IBCLCs in the group, such as Diana Cassar-Uhl, who would respond at the drop of a hat to any query I had.

Eli just turned one this month. We're still breastfeeding. He received only my expressed milk or breastfed from me until the day after he turned 11 months, apart from three small formula top ups in the early days post-delivery. He flat out refused to nurse for six weeks after that record breaking 11-month milestone, getting about one half to two thirds of his requirements from me until he fell ill with a nasty virus. During that virus, we reconnected with breastfeeding, and he now nurses one to four times a day from me, on his terms of course; never if I suggest it! He still has three bottles a day of formula. I've stopped pumping and my breasts are almost at the end of their marathon.

I have great love and support from my husband, of course, but he never could fully understand my emotional attachment to needing to feed, or provide any breast milk I could, along with the crazy hormones that come with it. To find others going through this, who you could connect with 24/7, really makes it feel like you have a whole bunch of people cheering you on ... who don't think you're going crazy either! I don't think I would have made it this far without their support, or without the help of those little snippets of info that made me realize something wasn't right with my son's tongue.

I think any mother who has had prior breast surgery for whatever reason would really benefit from widening her knowledge from the Internet, along with getting contacts in her local area who would be able to help her maintain a successful breastfeeding relationship, no matter how much milk she can produce. For basic breastfeeding advice on storing milk and expressing, the Australian Breastfeeding Association was really useful. Although health professionals, such as doctors and IBCLCs, are invaluable and have such a wide knowledge, sometimes things can be missed or their own beliefs (on things such as IGT or TT) can lead them to disregard treatment options. Being able to touch base with someone on the Web who has been through your issues can give you added advice or tips on where else to turn for a second opinion.

Amanda's Story

I still remember the first time I actually thought about breastfeeding. It was during a consultation for a breast reduction when I was 18. I had never had any reason to think about breastfeeding, though I knew what it was. I figured those gigantic mammary glands that I felt I had been cursed with must have some purpose, other than eliciting uncomfortable gawks from everyone I passed. My mother, who accompanied me to the appointment, asked the doctor how a reduction would affect breastfeeding. I remember thinking, "Who the hell cares. Just get them off my chest!" His response and practice, which I learned later is uncommon, was that he made every effort to spare the milk ducts. I even told my mom, "I'll just give formula." I will never forget the look of complete horror on her face, as if I'd planned to do my future, alleged child(ren) harm! She said, "You have no idea how much easier it is to nurse: in the middle of the night it's there, it's ready, it's warm, and it's easy and you get to hold your baby that much closer." And so the wheels began turning ... I had been breastfed, I learned, and being only 18 years old, and a fan of as much sleep as I could get, I figured that in the future I would nurse. Then I thought very little about the topic for 13 years ...

As soon as I learned I was pregnant, I delved into every ounce of reading material about babies, pregnancy, and breastfeeding I could find. I inundated my poor bystander husband with tidbits, facts, and a wealth of knowledge I could tell he cared little about. Engorgement, pain, pumping ... words that sent him into an alternate universe of thought, where I'm sure he thought about hunting, gathering, and all things masculine. He simply enjoyed the sight of the boobs I'd had reduced all those years ago, returning at a rapid pace to the size they were originally, before the surgery and before he knew them. I had some friends that nursed, but it was my best friend who passed on a lot of information about the importance of breastfeeding, both chemically and as a bonding time, through her experience. I figured I'd make sure I was successful by knowing what to expect at every stage. It was in a book I came across the line that, in effect said, "Women with a history of breast augmentation, particularly those who've had reductions, can expect to have issues nursing, if they are able to at all." It went on to describe that those with implants likely could, but the rest of us were—essentially—screwed. My heart sank. I was devastated, heartbroken, and mad at myself.

I was so married to the idea of breastfeeding, and was learning the benefits as it pertained to IQ, bonding, and immunity, when I came across that line. I decided I was a horrible mother; prenatally I'd already failed my child. A few days passed and I was determined that one line in one book could not be the end-all of the topic. I did what any sane, yet overly emotional pregnant woman would do: I turned to Google. As always, I got about a zillion hits, but many were unrelated and probably pornographic. Then I saw a link to a book on Amazon; the book was written by Diana West, IBCLC, specifically about breastfeeding after having a reduction, and the author's website, www.bfar.org (for BreastFeeding After Reduction) was mentioned as well. I ordered the book and ventured over to her website. Contrary to the one-line in the book that had rocked my world, it was an uplifting place with a plethora of information. There I found women who were successful in "BFARing", so much so that they were nursing toddlers.

For the next few months, I read everything, posted questions on the message board, and felt I was, at this point, qualified enough to attempt to BFAR with my own baby. There, I learned about goat's rue after 36 weeks, and after a breastfeeding class even met with a wonderful, angelic IBCLC who gave me a prenatal breastfeeding assessment. She saw I was already leaking colostrum and said, "Don't bother buying an SNS." Through the book by Diana West, I found references to the Facebook pages for Best for Babes and The Leaky Boob, and from there, the information I was exposed to exploded into a world of wonderful knowledge that is not readily discussed in any prenatal book.

Based on all that I read, I based my ideal birth plan on what would best support the breastfeeding relationship I desired. Unfortunately, having a natural hippy-esque birth, where my son magically exited my uterus without drugs and proceeded straight to skin on skin, did not happen. Due to my water breaking and my son deciding he wasn't ready to descend into the birth canal, I had to have a c-section and was mortified. Because I had expressed my breastfeeding concerns through the labor I endured for 26 hours, and because I was so lucky to have an obstetrician who is very pro-breastfeeding, she assured me as soon as he was born, if there were no complications, she'd place him skin to skin in the operating room—not the most common practice for an OB. Then, after I was all sewn up, we could resume skin to skin in recovery. That was precisely how our story played out.

My husband supported him to lay on my chest in the OR, and the little guy reached out and grabbed my nipple, making me realize babies are far more knowledgeable about what comes next than we give them credit for. He was rooting away, and once we were in recovery, my husband stripped him down and placed him on my skin and right to the boob he crawled. We were off. My husband, who apparently retained some of the vast amount of knowledge I heaped on him about breastfeeding, also told the nurses to please write on his little name sign, "No pacifiers. No bottles. Breastfed."

That first latch felt like success, and every latch thereafter, even when I was sore, reminded me I was doing it right. I continued to read the blogs, web pages, Facebook pages, and because of this I was ready and expecting the growth spurts, the days of endless nursing that just meant he needed me, not that I was a failure or wasn't producing enough. I turned to the Web when he was nursing four hours at a time, every night, only to learn I was, as I'd signed up to be, his pacifier, and that, "this too shall pass and you'll probably miss it." It was there I learned about supply and demand as it pertained to the commerce of my milk, not as any economics professor had ever explained. It was there I found thousands of women ready to give advice and say, "good job."

By the time I returned to work at 14 weeks postpartum, I had over 100 bags of milk ready to go. I pumped every chance I got, and I was going to convince my BFAR boobs I'd had triplets! I made sure my colleagues knew what I was doing, even to their shock and horror. (I'm a teacher so I have become a pro at pumping, and pumping quickly in various locations.) I can pump while driving, in closets, you name it!

The message boards, forums and blogs helped me learn that I was doing it right. I nursed on demand, co-slept, didn't introduce a bottle until I returned to work and threw any questions I had out into the blogs, message boards, and Facebook pages of groups I'd discovered while still pregnant. The support, answers, and tips I received helped to remind me that babies are not predictable, and that I was doing it right as long as I trusted my instinct. My son became a champion nurser, and I loved it. Our goal was to nurse for two years, though at 14 months he's just weaned himself. I already miss it, but as I'm five months pregnant, I will get to do it all over again soon enough. I'm sure my son was not a fan of nursing around my expanding belly, and the way my milk changed at 20 weeks was apparently no longer to his taste. He's discovered a world of solid food and organic DHA-supplemented milk, and we still have breast milk we defrost to get him through cold-and-flu season.

My vocabulary now includes words like "galactagogue," "colostrum," and "let-down," and I kind of enjoyed weirding people out when I nursed or talked about how long I nursed. I have directed pregnant friends and family to go to the sites and learn all they can from other moms, and to use the IBCLC services available at any number of local hospitals. I wish everyone had the support and access to support that I vigilantly sought out. I know that I gave my son everything he needs and will do so again in a few months for this little guy.

Kelly's Story

My breastfeeding journey began long before for my first pregnancy. I was 18 years old and a senior in high school. I would go on to have my first baby girl a full ten years later. I had a breast reduction when I just a child, still technically a teenager, when childbearing, let alone breastfeeding, was far, far from my mind. In retrospect, I don't recall the surgeon ever asking me any questions about my desire to breastfeed someday. At the time, I was so focused on what my breasts had done to me, I don't think I could have cared about what they would potentially do for my future children.

I went on enjoying life for the next ten years, never really thinking much about breastfeeding. I became an RN, fell in love with and married wonderful man, and had my first baby girl. During my pregnancy, I did take a breastfeeding class and read a little here and there, innocently hoping my breast reduction would cause no challenge for my baby and me. However, the birth didn't go quite how I envisioned. You see, being an RN, I suppose I trusted a little too much in the system. I ended up with a very healthy baby girl, born via c-section after many hours of labor, with both an epidural and Pitocin. As I was being wheeled into the operating room, I asked the doctors if I could have a vaginal birth next time. I spoke words that would take on new meaning in my life over the next few years.

My first baby girl, Dylan, nursed well, although we were challenged by tongue-tie, painful latch, my recovery from the cesarean, and, after a few days, a very unhappy, screaming baby. Our first night home from the hospital, as we attempted to slip into bed, she cried out over and over again after what seemed like a "good" feeding at the breast. Finally, I decided to supplement her, using a SNS, just the way the lactation consultant had shown me in the hospital. She was suddenly calm and resting. I was devastated. I knew then that things were not going as I had hoped. The next day I went to see the same LC who had seen us in the hospital and received some terrible advice. She took one look at my screaming baby, and told us that she was hungry and that my "hacked up" breasts were too much of a wild card. I was determined to give my baby breast milk, so I continued to comfort nurse for three months and pumped for a total of eight. It was an arduous journey. I'll never forget the disappointment I felt and the guilt that lingered.

Over the next two years, I spent countless hours working through my feelings and views on motherhood, and learning how I could personally improve the journey into life for my next baby. Still reeling from the cesarean birth, I found and joined my local ICAN chapter, and learned everything I could about VBAC (Vaginal Birth After Cesarean), natural childbirth, and how an early start to breastfeeding after an all-natural delivery ensured promising results for both mama and baby. I clung to every word that my mama friends told me who had had natural births and breastfed. I read and re-read websites, such as KellyMom, Breastfeeding Online, and BFAR/Low Milk Supply (www.lowmilksupply.org) to formulate my plan. I knew I would need to increase my milk supply should a new bundle of joy arrive again someday. As a result of my research, I began to think that a natural birth would dramatically improve my breastfeeding ability.

My local ICAN chapter started a Facebook group in addition to its monthly meetings. It became a place for women to go who were seeking facts, care provider information, and emotional support. I found myself on this page daily, sometimes more than once a day. Women were sharing their successes, and it was empowering. It enabled us to instantly connect when we did meet face to face because it had given us the opportunity to know each other. I also learned of VBACfacts.com, and found it a wonderful source of information. The creator of the page gave a talk locally that I was able to attend, and when I later wrote to her with some follow-up feedback and questions, we, too became Facebook friends. She has since started a closed Facebook group, VBAC Facts Community, which I turned to for increased online support.

About one month before my second daughter was born, after months of focusing on childbirth preparation and VBAC education, I got my mind back on breastfeeding. I suppose it was a beast I really didn't want to face. I re-read Diana West's book, *Defining Your Own Success: Breastfeeding After Reduction,* and I saw stories where women had similar experiences to mine. I continued to place so much of the blame from my first BFAR experience on my birth experience, and my previous lack of education. I continued to believe that I could "fix" any breastfeeding challenges if had my dream birth. I was excited, nervous, and ready.

After a picture-perfect labor and delivery of six short hours and only 21 minutes of pushing, my sweet Delilah was born. It was drug-free and everything I had envisioned. She came straight into my arms and never left me. Within 30 minutes of her birth, she nursed. The L&D nurse was so supportive during my delivery, but I'll never forget her words when I took my bra down to nurse the very first time. She saw my scars and matter-of-factly asked "did you nurse your first baby?" "Yes, of course," I said, begging to defend my situation. But to whom was I defending my story, her or myself?

I had the most incredible obstetrician, Dr. Damon Cobb. He fully supports what women want in their pregnancy and birth. He has gained quite the reputation for his support of VBAC and low-intervention births in general. Thankfully, Dr. Cobb "friends" his patients on Facebook, in an effort to make himself accessible for questions. He was unwavering in his positivity throughout my pregnancy. I communicated with him in those early days and weeks after Delilah was born, for continued support.

The first few days and weeks home with the new baby were fabulous. I was riding a birth high. I was a second-time mom and more confident than before. My milk had come in faster than it had after the cesarean, and though Delilah nursed round the clock, she seemed content. The first check-up after hospital discharge even showed a positive weight gain. As days turned into weeks, my curiosity and concern over her proper weight gain surfaced, and I began checking her weight weekly. A pattern soon emerged, and she was gaining about two-thirds of what a newborn should.

When the dust settled, it became clear that I would need to supplement. I came to the realization that the actual natural birth would not make a surgically-altered breast produce more milk, but it did give me the confidence to push through the tough months ahead. It allowed me to find strengths greater than I dreamt I had. When breastfeeding was tough again, I thought about my birth journey and what I had to overcome. I triumphed over some pretty tough odds, and breastfeeding for me became that parallel. I don't think other moms without the challenges I've had get off easy, so to speak, but some days I think that I appreciate my breastfeeding relationship just a little bit more deeply. It means the world to me. Each and every time my baby nurses, I remind myself just how far we have come. I could have given up countless times. With the help of friends who were always online, I was supported. No one goes along the same journey in life, but somehow the act of breastfeeding a baby is one where women just seem to understand. I met those women online. It was an almost daily mantra: you can breastfeed despite your surgery. Times were tough when the baby wasn't gaining as well as "normal," and I was afraid of the slippery slope of supplementing more. I had an unsupportive pediatrician who wanted me to immediately add formula to her diet. He had no idea where I had come from, my

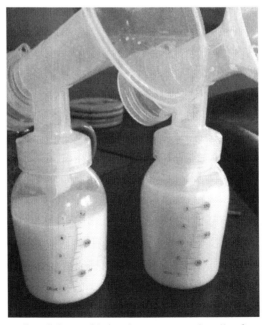

Kelly's labor of love: her pumped milk after returning to work when her daughter was six months old. —*Photo credit: Kelly Drzewiecki*

background, my passion, or where I was getting my support.

An online friend suggested I use Ask Dr. Sears (www.AskDrSears.com) as a resource for watching my baby's weight gain, wet and dirty diaper count, and overall nursing newborn guidance. Ultimately, I switched pediatric offices, and went to Sears Family Pediatrics in order to find more support. Dr. Bob Sears believed in me and naturally, supported my efforts. He encouraged me to keep breastfeeding, and helped me develop a supplementation schedule that would meet my baby's nutrition needs.

I also turned to Dr. Jack Newman for help, as his website is filled with some of the best breastfeeding videos I could find on the web. Dr. Newman even answered my personal emails. My very supportive husband got in on the action and wrote to Dr. Newman when we decided to give Motilium a try. I was already nursing round the clock, and pumping about five times a day, taking herbs and supplements. My baby was still not gaining quite enough—but we were so close! After much research, and a personal conversation via email with Dr. Newman about my background, he suggested giving it a go and recommended I order Motilium. I started taking the medicine as soon as it arrived, and I continued my schedule of nursing/pumping/supplementing. I noticed a definite increase in my production. I even got up to 250 ounces of milk in my freezer stash! I took pictures to remember it because I almost couldn't believe it. It was working! Still, I had moments of guilt and confusion. I was happy to be producing so much milk, but I felt sadness that it was medication-induced. I stayed on the Motilium for a few months and weaned off, very slowly.

A large decrease in my pump sessions meant less milk to use for supplementing, and we started dipping into that freezer supply around the time she was seven months old. By this time, I had far surpassed my own personal goals. I set tiny goals at first: make it to six weeks, then two, four, and six months. Once I hit the six-month goal, my next goal was to keep nursing when I went back to work, which I did. We are about a month away from her first birthday and if we make that goal, I'll be satisfied!

This past year has given me the greatest joy I have ever known. This was hard, hard work, but worth all the time and energy. My husband endured and supported my efforts, and for that I am forever thankful. We can chuckle now at some of the other adventures this special breastfeeding journey included: a broken freezer with milk melting before our eyes and a repair man being paid just to save the milk, a nursing strike, a pump-rental bill equivalent to a nice family vacation, a bottle of spilled milk that was cried over for very good reason, and an older sibling understanding that mama has to pump and that's just the way it is!

I can only hope that my daughters will not be faced with the challenges I had should they choose to breastfeed. If they need to consider a breast reduction someday, I will support their desires, but I will educate them on all the beautiful things breastfeeding has to offer. My vote would certainly be to wait until all their babies are fed.

Chapter 10

All Tied Up: Tongue Tie and Lip Tie

When my boys were born, I had never really heard of tongue tie and/or lip tie being an issue for babies. The more mamas I come to know and help support, the more often I hear about this condition, which, if left untreated, can end a breastfeeding relationship before it has time to become established. Babies with tongue and lip ties often have difficulty transferring adequate amounts of milk to meet their growing needs. Because they can't latch properly, nursing is extremely painful for the mother. When untreated, tongue and lip tie results in breast trauma (sore, cracked, and bleeding nipples).

As we know, for milk to be produced, it must be removed from the breasts—it's a sensitive system of supply and demand. If a mother doesn't have sufficient stimulation and adequate milk removal in the early days of breastfeeding, that can quickly take a toll on her supply, and ultimately end her breastfeeding journey. It is extremely important for long-term supply as well that mothers have a good start in the early weeks of breastfeeding, as this builds the prolactin receptor sites in the breasts, which are responsible for making sure she has enough milk when baby is three months old, six months old, and beyond. Tongue tie, if undiagnosed and/or untreated, will negatively affect breastfeeding in the short-term, as well as the long-term.

Thankfully, there are many online support groups for these mothers. Often, they have to advocate on their own behalf and seek out the correct treatment, rather than being directed in the proper way by healthcare professionals. We can only hope with increased awareness, and the growth of online-support communities, that solutions and care for these babies will become more readily available.

I remember the first mother that I ever helped with a tongue-tied baby. She was a friend and I offered to support her once her baby was born. I typically reach out to mothers right around the time their babies are due, or immediately postpartum, because that way when they need help, (and they most always do), they know they can easily call upon me. I was emailing and texting with my friend Jen, and she figured out pretty early on that her newborn was tongue-tied. She went through the necessary steps to get a referral from her pediatrician for a specialist to clip the tie, and in the meantime she dreaded and agonized over every feeding.

I remember when she was about a week out from her specialist's visit, she told me if she could just hang on for roughly 64 more feedings (yes, she had done the math and figured out the amount of physical suffering her breasts would endure in the next week), she'd be fine. As it turned out, she was able to get into the doctor's office shortly after our conversation, and was very relieved to know that help was so near. When she took her baby boy to the doctor, she was floored because the doctor refused to clip the tie. The doctor assumed her son's tongue-tie must not be "that bad" because the baby was gaining weight and was, therefore, obviously, transferring milk. Fearing for the longevity of their breastfeeding relationship, and knowing that things could not continue as they were, she flatly refused to leave the office without the procedure. Thankfully the doctor relented, performed the procedure, and sent them on their way.

I gave her after-care support that I found through the website of an IBCLC friend of mine, Fleur Bickford, and they were able to recover quickly and enjoy pain-free nursing sessions. Jen was very proactive about breastfeeding support from this point on. I referred her to The Leaky Boob on Facebook, and I would often see her there, posting questions and helping others with her experience. She didn't start out an advocate, but she ended up one, as did all of the mothers whose stories you'll read here.

Regina's Story

After a long, hard labor that left me exhausted and drained, our little firecracker was born. Aurora took a breath and screamed before her body was even born. That wail was the most pitiful thing I had ever heard. I reached down and grabbed her before the midwife could catch her and snuggled my sweet, still-wailing baby to my chest. She calmed down after a few minutes of wailing her heart out and realized that the world around her was new, and thus, exciting. So began our sweet, sensitive girl's life.

Within 30 minutes of giving birth, I attempted to nurse our baby. She wasn't very interested and started crying again when we tried to get her to latch. Since this was my first baby, and I only have a few memories of my mother breastfeeding my younger siblings, I assumed the difficulties were on my side. We soon learned otherwise. Aurora was tongue-tied. Thankfully, it was a classic tongue tie; nothing complicated. Her lingual frenulum was short and ran all the way up to the tip of her tongue and the very edge of her gum. Try as she might, she could not get her tongue to move the way it was supposed to to nurse properly, though she managed to get milk out, thankfully. Our midwife suggested we wait to see if the tongue tie would actually be a problem for nursing before exploring options for cutting it. I trusted her judgment and focused on learning to take care of my baby.

However, nursing continued to be difficult. Aurora was a very, very slow eater, and was frustrated with latching on. As for other new nursing pairs, the process was painful. I wasn't sure what was normal pain and what wasn't. I sought out advice from an online forum, and the only local person I knew of who would know about breastfeeding: a former La Leche League leader. She didn't have much help for me and didn't know any doctors who would cut the tongue tie. We consulted our daughter's doctor, and he said he wouldn't touch the tongue tie unless the baby wasn't gaining weight. I talked to my midwife, and she told me to limit the baby's nursing to ten minutes per side. I ignored this bit of bad advice, and to avoid using a nipple shield at all costs since that would, for sure, ruin my milk supply (this is bad advice, too, but I unfortunately believed her on this one).

By the time Aurora was two weeks old, nursing was torture. The pain was getting worse. Every feeding felt like the baby was tearing my nipples apart. My nipples started splitting and bleeding. I had to wake my husband up during the nights to help me force myself to nurse our wailing baby. The baby nursed for 45 minutes to an hour every feeding, and ate every one and a half hours to every two hours. Those early weeks with our sweet Aurora are a blur of pain and tears for me. I refused my husband's offers to get me bottles and formula because I felt like I would be a failure as a mother if I didn't breastfeed my baby.

Finally, I shared my struggles in detail on a forum where I had found information in other areas to be trustworthy. How I stumbled upon this particular forum is a wonder to me. It is filled with highly educated women, college professors, mothers, doctors, nurses, and women who care about research and truth—and there were several La Leche League leaders, and at least one International Board Certified Lactation Consultant (IBCLC) at any time. They took my pitiful story and helped me find help. They gave me links to websites (KellyMom and LLLI were especially helpful), explained what kind of procedure Aurora was in need of, gave me ideas for reducing the pain, and soothed my fears about using a nipple shield. They listened to my tortured posts, and shared their stories of pain and success. They encouraged me and helped as best they could. That help was what made the difference for me.

Finally, after four weeks of struggling with the torture of feeding my daughter, I took action. I called over a dozen doctors of various kinds and sent my husband on an early-morning run to buy a nipple shield. At long last, I felt a bit of hope. My daughter was no longer tearing my nipple off and breastfeeding was less painful. It was still painful, and it would take weeks for my nipples to heal, but it was no longer quite as awful. The search for a doctor who would listen to me was difficult. We finally found a pediatric surgeon in the city an hour away who would perform the surgery—for $800 plus a $90 office visit beforehand. We didn't have insurance, were fresh out of college, and were saddled with huge debt. We knew we couldn't pay that, and that using nipple shields long term would be less expensive.

At my six-week check-up, my midwife clicked her tongue at the nipple shield, and finally decided she would make a few phone calls to some doctors she knew. The ladies on the forum had encouraged me to be pushy since medical professionals can often get more information from other medical professionals than I could just by calling their offices. Sure enough, by the end of my check-up, the midwife had received a response from a doctor I had already called—he was willing to look at the tongue tie and cut it in his office if he felt it was warranted.

One glance in the mouth was all it took. It was a thin, simple tongue-tie, so no cauterizing or anesthesia would be needed. Two snips from the scissors was all it took to free my daughter's tongue. She wailed at being held down for the procedure, and there was a tiny drop of blood when I picked her up to nurse her. She latched on easily and nursed for several minutes before pulling away calm and happy.

I continued to use the nipple shield for several weeks while my nipples healed. It took about ten weeks before nursing was pain-free. The tears in my nipples healed, and I stopped using the shield. I continued to experience shooting pains for several months, likely from nerve damage. Even today, though, I have a reminder of those tough times: one of my nipples remains scarred from the damage that was done to it four years ago.

Melissa's Story

My second child was born at home, as planned, and as her brother Adam was about two and a half years earlier. With Adam, I had extremely painful nipples for about two weeks—I cried during and iced between feedings. I had read so many books, and I had been to La Leche League meetings. Looking back, I have no idea why I didn't reach out for help! He was colicky from three weeks to four months, which made motherhood very difficult, and contributed to my postpartum depression (PPD). As well, he was terribly "spitty" until around his first birthday, but we nursed and we loved it. Well, we loved it until I was a couple months pregnant with Leah. He was past the age of two by then, and we did what we could to get both our needs met as much as possible—including night weaning and cutting back. He still nurses occasionally, but not regularly anymore.

Leah was born at 40 weeks, after less than two hours of labor— the midwives just made it! Leah went straight to me, and we were covered with warm towels for hours. It was lovely. We didn't even know she'd left a huge poop on me until we unwrapped her for the newborn exam three hours after she was born. She wasn't interested in latching immediately, but an hour postpartum She latched, and nursed frequently from then on. I noticed right away that she did not open her mouth very wide to latch, but I figured we'd work on it. I had read all the stuff about laid-back breastfeeding/Biological Nurturing, so many of our first pictures were of me trying to guide her onto the breast that way. By the time she was a day old, my nipples were bleeding and scabbing. It was painful, but this time I was not going to white-knuckle through it. I had found my support system, a local mom's group where I live, and I knew exactly who to call. I called my friend from the group who is an IBCLC, and set up a home visit on Monday afternoon, when Leah was just 48 hours old. Kate came over, her own three-week-old baby in tow, and observed and examined us both. A quick oral exam found a posterior tongue tie. She advised some position changes, and the use of coconut oil for my nipples, which helped immediately with the pain and damage.

We carried on, but it was not easy nor was it fun. There was just something that was off. I knew that was a problem with nursing because nursing had become pretty much effortless with Adam after the first few weeks. I knew exactly what I was missing, and it made me sad. Leah would not open her mouth wide. She pursed her lips like a little bird and slurped the nipple in. Not that she could hold it for very long anyway. She was pulling on the nipple, curling her chin to her chest, popping off, etc. It took forever to get through a feeding, though luckily she was transferring plenty and stayed on her 95% curve. I felt like I should be able to fix it. I had read so much on the subject. I am going through the comprehensive course to become a Volunteer Breastfeeding Counselor with Breastfeeding USA. I had a beautiful nursing relationship with my son for years. Why couldn't I fix this?

We continued to have problems, and I continued to receive help via email from Kate. She was willing to refer us to the local children's hospital Ear, Nose and Throat (ENT) practice. I was having a hard time weighing the pain and risks of surgery and anesthesia against possible improvement. I decided for the moment that we'd done as much as we could, and we'd just struggle. After the first days, I didn't have many nursing photos, and none in which I was not frowning. I am not shy about nursing in public, but it was nearly impossible to do, keeping up with an almost-three-year-old, and trying to keep my baby latched long enough to get some milk, then dealing with the inevitable projectile vomit. I didn't know what to do. You don't get much sympathy (outside of lactation consultants) when you have a feeding problem, yet an abundant milk supply and a fat baby.

Kate,
Help me, please :) I swear, If I didn't believe that breastfeeding is necessary for normal development I'd quit right now.

I need to bring her in to you. I think there's something wrong with Leah and/or I'm still having a forceful letdown issue. Nursing her is miserable about 90% of the time. Don't get me started on what it's like out of the house with her pulling off and crying every 3 sucks. I've stopped all pumping hoping to get supply down, but she's smacking and gagging and pulling off even with a soft empty breast. Sometimes on the right breast she can projectile vomit after a very short time nursing. I feel so freaking sorry for her when it happens when we're nursing lying down and she ends up with barf in her eyes, ears, and hair. I almost feel cruel for breast-feeding her. I'm scared to give a pacifier thinking she will be so happy to have a nipple that doesn't hose her that she'll refuse the breast after.
/whine

Tomorrow I have lots of appointments (midwife at 11 and CST for Leah at 2) but Thursday until about 3 and all of Friday are open, and next week, too.

~Melissa

Melissa's desperate email to her friend Kate, an IBCLC, who referred her to a tongue-tie specialist.

I remember how I found the Tongue Tie Babies Support Group (TTBSG) on Facebook. A mother had posted a question on the Analytical Armadillo Facebook page (www.facebook.com/TheAnalyticalArmadillo), and her symptoms sounded similar to Leah's. I posted some things that had worked for us—the probiotics and digestive enzymes, the elimination diet, the frequent burping, etc, and our decision not to do a revision of the tongue tie. A page administrator of Analytical Armadillo posted in response to me something like, "Yes, you can work around tongue tie or you can address the tongue tie." I was stung. I can still remember how it felt. It threw me into a tailspin of self-doubt—was I doing the right thing for my baby? Was I denying her care that she needed? Was I just lazy and taking the path of least resistance? Add that to the sleep deprivation of a baby who couldn't sleep without being burped and/or spitting up frequently, and I turned into a late-night mama on a mission. With my smart phone in hand, I researched tongue tie from my bed!

I started doing more research on Leah's condition, starting with the Analytical Armadillo's blog (www.analyticalarmadillo.co.uk) and

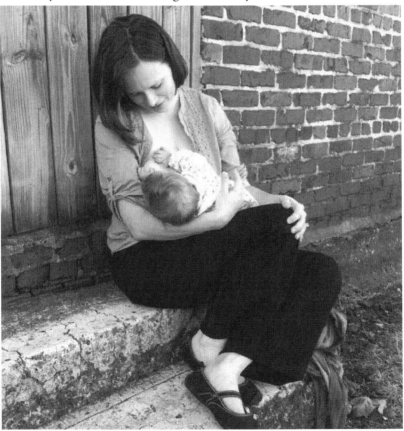

Melissa finally nursing comfortably in public about six weeks post tongue-tie procedure. —*Photo credit: Melissa Cline*

other places online. I emailed dentists in the area who advertised laser revision, and sadly, no one ever contacted me. I read story after story of moms and babies just like us. I read success stories and "we're on our third revision and my baby still isn't breastfeeding" stories. I read the articles on Dr. Kotlow's web page (www.kiddsteeth.com). I learned that tongue tie and lip tie often go together, and discovered Leah's lip tie myself. No wonder she couldn't flange her top lip: it was tightly tied. I posted photographs to the page, and page administrators, many of them experienced IBCLCs, and other mamas commented on what they saw. I read that anesthesia and the risk it entails was not necessary with laser revision by an experienced doctor or dentist. I read about the potential long-term consequences of untreated tongue tie. I felt intense regret that I didn't know about this sooner, and wondered if Adam's "colic" was related to his tongue and lip ties, which are pretty obvious looking in his mouth. I talked with my husband about traveling to a provider on the TTBSG recommended list as they vett providers, and maintained a list of those who are using best practices and/or have a good track record for results. I asked question after question on the Facebook page.

The closest recommended providers were both a five-hour drive away, and the thought of doing that alone with an eleven week-old baby was horrifying, so I looked into taking an airplane. My husband's work travel had racked up some frequent-flyer miles that would take care of a plane ticket to the most experienced provider on the list, and our health savings account would cover the surgery. All we'd need to pay out of pocket would be the hotel and rental car. The next business day, I called Dr. Kotlow's office to talk about scheduling an appointment. They were very kind and said they'd work around the flights I could get. Nine days after starting the real search for info about tongue-tie, I was on a plane with my daughter on our way to New York.

From the airport, we went straight to the dental office. The revision went well, and she was out of my arms a mere ten minutes, just as promised. Dr. Kotlow demonstrated the stretching we would need to do to prevent reattachment, and we checked in at our hotel, ate, and drove to an IBCLC consult with Norma Ritter, one of the

TTBSG members who commented on Leah's photos, who was about 45 minutes away. Also, I met in the waiting area an administrator from the Facebook page who was there for a repeat revision for her daughter. It helped me feel less alone.

The TTBSG page maintains a document of best practices aftercare for tongue-tie revision. It talks about bodywork (chiropractor/CST/osteopathy), and the importance of bodywork in releasing restriction caused by the ties. It includes homeopathy for pain relief and healing, and links to videos of how to stretch. I can't imagine how I would have felt walking in for the surgery without that detailed plan in hand. It was also reassuring to know that I'd have all those mamas and volunteers at my fingertips after the revision. Honestly, the aftercare was traumatic for me, as well as my baby, and it helped me stay sane to be able to vent and ask questions about my technique and my daughter's reaction to the stretching (and the recommended Rescue Remedy helped us both). There are even mamas on the page who have had their own tongue-ties revised and could talk about how it felt.

We flew home the next day and continued with recommended

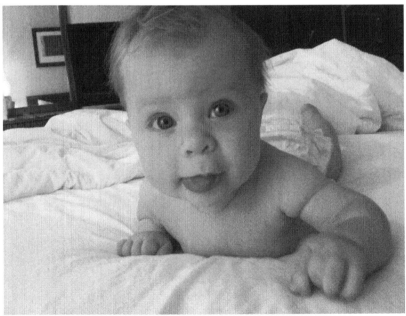

Leah, showing off her un-tied tongue. —*Photo credit: Melissa Cline*

aftercare. We were fortunate to find not one, but three craniosacral therapists (CST) who worked with children. The decrease in air swallowing was immediately apparent. Other habits took longer to unlearn, and continued IBCLC and CST visits helped. The first CST session after the revision was so awesome. We had the best nursing session of her life after it! We continued to see improvement for the next two months, with the CST helping immensely. I did the stretching aftercare for about twice as long as the dentist recommended. I turned to the group once again at about eight weeks post-revision when I noticed her tongue seemed restricted again, and got some suggestions on how to reopen at home with gentle pressure.

Things are very different now: we can nurse out and about, we can nurse in a carrier, and no longer must I tow spit rags around everywhere. Even still, almost three months later, I sometimes cry with joy looking down and seeing her big fish lips latch. I have posted several sappy "thank you" messages to the TTBSG page. I don't know what I would have done otherwise. Would I have gone to the local ENTs and put her through anesthesia, more pain compared to laser (they use the more painful methods of scissors and cautery), and who knows what they recommend for aftercare? Would I have tried the extra work of pumping and bottle-feeding, as my husband suggested (out of love, and out of the ubiquitous cultural belief that bottle-feeding is somehow easier)? Would I have had a lifetime of regret over weaning early or not enjoying nursing her? I'm glad I don't have to find out, and as called out and criticized as I felt at that Analytical Armadillo response, it sent me in the direction I needed to go to save my nursing relationship.

Kim's Story

I wasn't prepared to experience pain with breastfeeding after the birth of my second son. I took for granted that already going through myriad latch issues with my first son and the subsequent trips to a lactation consultant trained me to know how to beat any issues for a second child, and counted as "paying my dues" in the breastfeeding department.

It was the second day after my son's uneventful and wonderful homebirth that I started feeling raw and sore. His latch seemed perfect to me, but something was definitely wrong. It was confusing and heartbreaking to think of facing another struggle. I took my issue to Twitter, explaining that we were experiencing pain and blistering. Immediately I received several tweets in reply asking if my son was "tongue tied."

I had heard of this, but never gave it any thought. I even recall my midwife looking into my son's mouth, and not saying anything about his tongue being "tied." I looked for myself, and underneath his tongue I immediately noticed the frenulum had his tongue "tied" very close to the bottom of his mouth, and his tongue was shaped like an adorable little heart. Both were very real signs of tongue tie.

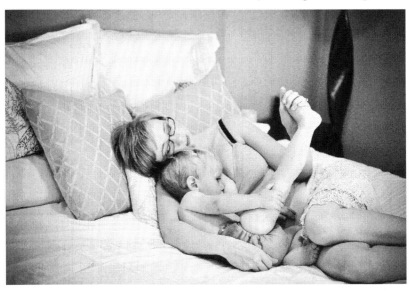

Kim and her son still enjoying breastfeeding more than two years after having his tongue tie procedure. —*Photo credit: Kim Rosas*

I fielded responses on Twitter, and went back and forth with several mothers, even a few IBCLCs, who suggested I take him to our pediatrician who could hopefully clip the frenulum. Without clipping we could run into several issues, pain being one, and a drop in supply for me if he was not nursing correctly, which could lead to weaning or supplementing. I fully intended to nurse my baby for as long as possible. Even though I was afraid of inflicting what I assumed would be a painful experience onto my two-day-old baby, I made the call.

Our pediatrician confirmed the tongue tie, but wasn't allowed to cut it. We were referred to an Ear, Nose, and Throat specialist, who also confirmed and rated it a "3 out of 4" in severity. A local anesthetic was applied, and in two seconds his frenulum was cut. I waited outside of the door; my fresh mama hormones couldn't bear to see him in pain, so my husband held him. At the sound of his cry, I ran in, dropped by bra cup, and latched him, bloody mouth and all.

The difference in his latch was immediate. I could tell his latch was deeper and that the tongue could extend properly. He happily nursed for a few minutes and calmed down; I was relieved that we had made the right decision. I thanked the friends on Twitter who offered me guidance and suggested my son might be tongue-tied, which we corrected early enough to prevent even more pain and a possible problem with our nursing relationship. I wrote about our tongue-tie experience on my own blog, and have seen many mothers receive answers to their questions from finding the post through search engines.

My son is now almost two and a half years old, and we are still nursing. I don't know that we could have overcome his severe tongue tie without clipping, and who knows how long it would have taken for our pediatrician to notice? After reading stories of women nursing through pain for months before receiving the news, I am truly grateful that there are women on Twitter, message boards, Facebook, and writing on blogs who can guide new mothers and offer support. It is important to realize that not every woman is an expert, and that all advice should be taken with a grain of salt; if merited, the guidance you receive online should be followed up with a visit to a midwife, doctor, or preferably an IBCLC.

Chapter 11

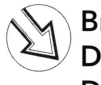 **Breastfeeding with Depression and Mood Disorders**

The Internet has the amazing ability to keep us from feeling truly isolated, even when we might be physically isolated. I know that was my experience—I reached out to find like-minded friends in a new area where I had recently moved, and with a few clicks, I found a group of women with whom I would have loved to have coffee dates and picnics in the park!

For new mothers who are suffering from depression, the Internet is often a lifeline. It offers them help and support that they often cannot find in their daily lives. Have you ever had someone ask how you are, more out of politeness than genuine interest, and five minutes later you realized you are still rambling on, when all they really wanted to hear was, "I'm fine, thanks for asking?"

The work that mothers do is tough. It is physically and emotionally exhausting, and the schedule is relentless. Becoming a mother changes who we are forever. It changes us physically, and it changes our daily lives. If you give up your career to stay home, you have some major adjustments to get used to. If you stay on the career track and opt to place your child in another person's care, then you likely have stress or sadness about that choice too. There are the financial strains of parenthood, and it can completely change your relationship with your partner. Did I mention that your old favorite jeans you wore before becoming a mother might not fit anymore, so your self-image may be tangled up in the metamorphosis of you as "mom?"

Given all these tremendous changes, it is no surprise that some mothers get depressed. You might experience depression for the first time in the postpartum period, and have difficulty recognizing it. Or, you might have suffered from depression for years, and pregnancy and motherhood have amplified those emotions, making it very difficult to cope. Of course, the Internet can't cure depression, but it can help you feel less isolated and direct you to sources of support. There are many resources available for new mothers battling depression—if you are struggling, please reach out for help. You might see yourself in these stories, or they will help you become more aware of mothers you meet who are suffering. All of these women found support online, and it was breastfeeding that brought them to the Internet in search of answers.

Devona's Story

We almost didn't make it. My daughter, Olivia, was five weeks old, and I almost gave up on breastfeeding because it just felt like the cards were stacked against us. I sat in my glider in the living room of our dinky apartment, letting her painfully gnaw on my nipple in the middle of the night, while I alternated singing hymns for comfort and sobbing in despair. I wondered if she'd ever sleep through the night. I wondered why it made my toes curl with pain every time she latched on. I wondered why she spit up forcefully so often, and was she keeping any of my milk down? Was there something wrong with my milk? Maybe everyone was right and we were too young to have a baby. Maybe this was a big mistake. My husband Rob and I were just 22 and 23, respectively. Ironically, the one thing I never wondered was if I had postpartum depression.

In spite of my best research, I had a terrible birth. I had consented to an induction I didn't want, which turned into an epidural I didn't want, and a traumatic birth, which left me feeling like a failure. It was already a huge blow to my confidence, which wasn't very strong to begin with, and I was so worried that I would fail at breastfeeding too. Because Rob and I were so young, we didn't have any friends with kids. We hardly even had any married friends. I had no one to turn to in the real world for advice. I didn't know it at the time, but the depression was isolating me from everyone, even my husband. Rob worked long hours at a newspaper, so I would struggle to make dinner for myself, feed the baby, and keep myself on a schedule. When he came home, I would act as if nothing was wrong, but the days blurred into one, and I felt like I never got out of my nursing spot in that glider. The Internet was the only place I felt comfortable reaching out.

Rob and I kept a blog, called *Love and Blunder* (www.loveand-blunder.com), where we shared our parenting dreams and fears with a small but devoted following. One of our readers invited me to join a website for naturally minded moms, called Gentle Christian Mothers (www.gentlechristianmothers.com), or GCM, because she could tell I was struggling. I logged in the first time, and I instantly felt like I was at home. Instead of "bothering" Rob with my difficulties, I would open up a browser page, and click away onto the pages of GCM. "Help! I think I'm failing, and it hurts really bad when she latches, and I'm worried I'm turning her into a bad sleeper because I can't get her to stay asleep longer than an hour or two."

"Oh my gosh, do I remember those days!" someone would reply. "You can't feed a baby too much! Hang in there!" I just needed someone to tell me it was okay that I had a hard time getting my infant back to sleep, or to give me links to the La Leche League website articles, which explained normal infant behavior, because I was always so sure I was making mistakes. I also needed women to give me permission to make mistakes, as it was really reassuring to hear someone say, "Oh, I would do things so differently now! I accidentally did something-or-other, and somehow, it all turned out okay. You'll get the hang of it."

As Olivia grew and developed, I also grew more confident. The advice I got on GCM helped me to fix small latch problems so nursing no longer hurt, and I became more self-assured. I found support in introducing solids gently, and Olivia was not only growing, but thriving! I started to feel like I might actually be a decent mother—maybe even a good one—even if my daughter still needed to nurse for a long time to fall asleep. I started opening back up to my husband, and feeling more secure when we were out and about. When we hit the milestone of nursing until one year, I jumped for joy! I had initially set the goal of nursing until she was six months, and we had made it twice that far, and we weren't even planning on weaning yet! I was almost back to my normal self as Olivia turned 15 months old. When I got those two pink lines again, Rob and I were determined to have a better birth experience on the second go-around. My online mamas advised me to find a midwife, which was one of the best choices I ever made.

My second daughter, Elise, was born in the water, and started breastfeeding right away. With my experience parenting Olivia, I knew it was no big deal to nurse her to sleep, and to feed her whenever she seemed hungry. I can't be sure if it was the more positive birth experience or the better support system, but I didn't suffer from depression after my second birth. I even got the courage to reach out to my "real life" support system, and joined our local La Leche League group, where I learned even more about the breastfeeding relationship and biology. Before I knew it, I had gone from a mom desperately seeking out help at three in the morning to the mom offering the support to the women coming up behind me!

During my third pregnancy, a group of friends and I started moderating a private Facebook group for naturally minded mothers. It is one of many Facebook groups just like it. One thing I've learned, having been on both the giving and receiving end of support, is that the questions new moms have are almost always the same. I have asked, "How often should my six-month-old be nursing at night?" I have offered the answer to the same question more than a dozen times to a dozen different moms. I have shared my personal cure for mastitis—cabbage leaves—in a support thread, which has also included the advice to nurse on the affected side first, use a warm compress, and hand express in the shower, at least as many times. It's encouraging to me. Eight years ago I started out asking these questions, and now I have seen the next group of women grow from seeker to advisor.

We used to live in small communities where we parented alongside our neighbors, sisters, and best friends. Now, we parent alone in our homes, never seeing another person struggling with things that are common and easily fixed, often just with the kind words of, "you can do it!" The Internet has given us back that community. It has also added the benefit of constant access to support. The immediate feedback is so beneficial when you're dealing with a real problem, and someone can be that voice encouraging you to head to the lactation consultant or pediatrician, even if just for some advice on whether you should nurse your baby once more. I don't know what would have happened to me if I hadn't been able to find community at 2 a.m. Your very best friend in the world is not going to want you knocking at that hour, looking for advice, but someone, somewhere is definitely going to be online to answer your questions for you. Even if they can't answer it, they can at least offer you a virtual hug and let you know they've been there too.

Andrea's Story

I don't remember making the decision to breastfeed. I had always felt that it was the right thing to do even though my sister and I were not breastfed, and I cannot recall being exposed to breastfeeding mothers while growing up. I suffer from environmental allergies and allergy-induced asthma, and when I was pregnant with my oldest child, I read research that stated that breastfeeding would give my baby the best possible advantage health-wise, particularly for allergies and asthma, which just solidified my resolve. However, despite my strong feelings, I didn't read much about breastfeeding before giving birth, in books or online. I assumed—as many women must do—that it would be an intuitive act, something that you just do with minimal thought.

I am American, but I have lived in a small city in the United Arab Emirates for the past eight and a half years. I have two children, a boy and a girl, who were both born by c-section in a hospital here. They are four years apart, and their breastfeeding relationships with me have been quite different. My relationship with my first child, Laith, was complicated and filled with anguish and sadness for the first several months. In contrast, my daughter and I successfully breastfed from the moment I put her to my breast. Moreover, because I was in good mental health after her birth, I did not experience the torment and stress that I did with my son, nor did I require even a fraction of the help I needed with him.

At 38 weeks into my pregnancy with Laith, I went into labor and ended up having a c-section due to continuous bleeding that indicated a ruptured placenta. I had planned on having an un-medicated, natural birth, so needless to say, I was rather disappointed by my son's entry into this world. I was not given him right away per hospital policy, something I had not thought to ask about during my prenatal visits (the hospital claims to follow the American system, in which babies delivered by c-sections not involving general anesthesia are given to their mothers immediately following birth. I assumed I would be afforded the same rights). It wasn't until approximately four or five hours later, after he had spent some time under the bili lights for jaundice, that I got to meet him for the first time.

Those first hours with Laith are rather fuzzy. I remember trying to breastfeed him once he was given to me, and being wholly unsuccessful. He rooted around and tried to grab onto my nipple, but I could not get him to latch on. This scenario repeated itself at each successive attempt to feed him for the duration of my hospital visit. Each time, after five to ten minutes of futile effort, he would fall back asleep and I would give up, unsure of what to do to help him. I kept thinking that the next time we tried, it would all fall into place and I would think, "Ah, yes, this is just how nature intended it!" I repeatedly asked the nurses, who alleged to be trained lactation consultants, for help. They spoke to me a little condescendingly and, even though they could not get Laith to latch either, assured me that we would "get it" very soon. They would exit the room briskly, leaving me to wonder what the hell was wrong with me.

After four days, I was released from the hospital. As we stepped through the door of our apartment, panic overwhelmed me. I was now alone and completely responsible for the feeding of this small creature—and I physically could not do it! Fortunately, despite the PPD-induced haze, I managed to grasp the importance of pumping milk in order to keep my supply up, and to have on hand for future bottle-feedings when I had to return to my job as an English as a Second Language instructor at a nearby university. When feeding after feeding failed, I filled bag after bag with milk, wondering if my son was getting anything at all.

One week passed from his birth, and Laith was listless when awake, always fidgeting and rooting around. When he slept, he slept like a rock, and keeping him awake for feedings was proving an impossible task. We had been advised to try feeding him with a dropper and cup as the hospital was very pro-breastfeeding and never once mentioned formula as an option. However, he was getting so little from them, and I couldn't tell if he was getting anything from me, so we headed back to the hospital. We learned that he had lost weight–perhaps a little more than he should have—but seemed fine otherwise, and we were again sent home with the words, "Keep trying. It will all work out soon."

I began to really despair at this point. Clearly, my son wasn't getting enough nourishment, but no one seemed willing or able to deal with it. The only LCs I knew of were the women in the hospital where I had given birth, and they hadn't been any help at all. I had no mother friends who had dealt with breastfeeding issues and could offer suggestions. One local mother of four children learned of my troubles and offered to come and see what my problem was, but she said the same thing as the hospital staff: relax and keep trying. It was extremely frustrating and disheartening.

I should mention that my journey with breastfeeding was also complicated by the fact that I was suffering from postpartum depression. Really, it was just a continuation of the mostly untreated depression I had been experiencing for 13 years prior to having a child, but the hormonal changes after birth gave my debilitating emotional state a new depth and form that I had never experienced before. Throughout my regular attempts at breastfeeding Laith, I cried continuously. The tears seemed to have no end. While I was spared the horror of wishing harm to my newborn, I did daydream regularly about running away to a place where no one would find me. I imagined myself packing my bags and stealing out the front door in the middle of the night. In short, I felt trapped by the small person in my arms, and I was resentful towards him for that.

Nine days after Laith's birth, another friend came to visit me. As I cried to her about my inability to properly breastfeed Laith, and my general failure as a new mom, she took a look at him and told me to go get a bottle and fill it with my pumped milk. I had been admonished by the hospital to not give bottles under any circumstances, but because I was greatly concerned and out of ideas, I took her advice. I felt sick to my stomach as I watched my hungry son suck the milk from the bottle in a matter of a few minutes. My child had been near-starving! Luckily, I also realized that feeding pumped milk in a bottle was a better alternative to formula, and so we began a bottle and breastfeeding routine that took up a significant portion of each day.

I had heard about La Leche League International (LLLI) during my pregnancy from a few moms and somehow in the fog of depression that enveloped me, I remembered that resource and decided I should see if I could contact them by email to get some help. I found their online forums, and began to "lurk," looking at different posts about feeding newborns. Not long after, I created an account and submitted a request to be matched with an online LLL leader for individual support.

Between the forum and the anonymous leader I was matched up with, I managed to finally obtain effective breastfeeding advice. I would submit questions to the LLL leader, and she would respond within 12 hours. I asked about working on latch, supply issues (I ended up with overactive letdown and oversupply, probably exacerbated by the constant pumping), sleeping issues as they relate to breastfeeding, and other topics. I posted regularly on the forum about my concerns, and received assurances and feedback from other mothers who had found themselves in the exact same position with their newborns. It was really wonderful!

I joined two other forums shortly after creating an account at LLLI, and those websites/forums also provided valuable breastfeeding information, but I did not have the free time to devote to a major presence on either of them, and because I had chosen LLLI first, I tended to be loyal to this group. Additionally, I would look up breastfeeding information online and came across a few blogs (blogging was really becoming popular around the time Laith was born) through Google searches, but the forums were my main source of support and knowledge. I feel fortunate to have chosen such a reputable source of breastfeeding knowledge right from the start. There is a lot of information available online for newly breastfeeding moms, and it isn't all accurate or even valuable.

Because I was depressed, I stayed home a lot with my son during his first year. Getting him ready to go out, and preparing the things I needed to do so seemed an insurmountable task much of the time, so I simply didn't leave the house unless I had to. As a result, I began to spend increasing amounts of time on the Mother-to-Mother forums, where I enjoyed getting to know other mothers more intimately, and discussing the various aspects of breastfeeding and mothering.

La Leche League affected all areas of my breastfeeding relationships with both of my children. For example, I might have weaned my son earlier had I not met such a large group of women who were breastfeeding their children well into the toddler years and beyond. It was considered so normal, such an important part of a child's development, that my attitude towards extended breastfeeding went from one of distaste to a feeling like I was part of an elite group, to one where I hardly gave any thought to how "different" I was compared to the average mother. I don't think I would have arrived at this place had I not been surrounded, in a virtual sense, by other women practicing the same thing.

Today, I still call many of these mothers I met online my friends. In fact, some of them probably know more details about certain aspects of my life than my friends in real life. I have never met any of them, as I've been halfway around the world and have had little opportunity to do so, but I can say that I would not have breastfed as successfully, or for as long, without their aid and concern.

When I think back to that time nearly six years ago, I'm not really sure where the determination to exclusively breastfeed came from. I'm fairly certain—and I don't mean this in a holier-than-thou way, but simply as a cause for curiosity–that most new mothers in my shoes would have turned to formula. I do know that my breastfeeding relationship with my son would not have flourished without the availability of the Internet. Without my online window to valuable insight and wisdom from trained breastfeeding experts and experienced breastfeeding mothers, I might have been an exclusively pumping mother or I might have turned to formula, believing I had no other options.

Bess's Story

When my oldest daughter was ten months old, I found out I was pregnant again. I was terrified and nervous that my supply would disappear, or that nursing would become painful and she would be forced into weaning. I bought a book on tandem nursing and devoured the information. I continued to breastfeed her through my entire pregnancy, and it went better than I expected. Sometimes, the moment she latched on was a little painful, but I was comfortable for the most part. My supply dropped a lot but was never completely eliminated. Though she did ask to nurse less frequently, she never stopped wanting to nurse. When she was 19 months old, I gave birth to my second daughter. After reading so many amazing stories on tandem nursing, I was excited and ready to take on the challenge! I thought it would be the best bonding experience ever, and I would love every second of it.

It didn't go as planned, though. We were under a lot of stress. When my second daughter was only ten days old, we made a huge move 900 miles back to our home state, then lived with my mom for two months while we got settled and looked for our own place. I started getting angry easily. My mood would wildly swing from one direction to the other. I felt out of control, and I felt panicked by my feelings and behavior. I told everyone that I wasn't suffering from postpartum depression, because I didn't feel depressed. I wondered if I was crazy, though, because I was getting mad so easily. And not just at anyone. I was getting angry at my oldest daughter, my sweetheart, especially when she nursed. When she would nurse I felt my blood pressure rise, and I'd be overtaken with this unexplainable, unprovoked rage. I felt like I wanted to smack her face off my breast. I would sit there and not move until I felt like I couldn't take another second, and then tell her her time was up. The entire time she nursed her eyes would wearily stare at me, like I was bomb about to go off. She could sense my anger radiating off of me. She stayed away from me a lot more, and began to act out around me more often. She only wanted me when she wanted to nurse, and I became sad and bitter over the entire experience. Three months after my second daughter was born, whom I never felt this anger towards while nursing, we moved into our own place. The craziness of the move kept us so busy that three days passed before I realized that my oldest had not asked to nurse in that time. I decided to go with it, and the few times she asked to nurse in that week I told her it was not time yet and just like that, she stopped asking and she never breastfed again.

After the move and her weaning, we healed and I stopped feeling angry. Our relationship began to mend, though it took a full year before I felt we were close again, and a full two years for me to come to a place of forgiveness for my own behavior. I still have so much guilt and wish I could go back in time and redo things—somehow get some kind of control of myself and to really do tandem nursing right, without the crazy hormones and the touched-out feelings that came with them.

It wasn't until much later that I discovered something called post-partum mood disorder (PPMD). It's not depression like PPD, but wild, unexplained mood swings. I was reading about the description of the disorder, and it fit me to a T. When I became pregnant with my third daughter, I was terrified of what would happen if I tried to tandem nurse again. My second daughter ended up self-weaning during pregnancy, so I never found out. I was simultaneously sad and relieved.

I tell moms about my story sometimes, but I always let them know that this is the rare exception. I've read so many tandem nursing stories, and none of the ones I've read have been like mine. I was the one bad experience out of a sea of wonderful, blessed stories. I beg them not to make a decision to wean based on what I went through, but if they tandem and are having bad thoughts and feelings, they can come to me because I have experienced that before.

Through the entire three months that I was struggling with tandem nursing, I would leak out on Twitter that tandem nursing wasn't going well. I never said to what extent because I had such guilt and felt so horrible about my own thoughts and feelings towards my daughter, but I received so much support. Many people jumped in to give me advice and tips on how to manage nursing her, such as giving her certain activities to distract her when nursing the baby, or setting a timer for when she nursed. None of it was a cure for what we were experiencing, but it was so nice to just get that kind of support from other moms and know that I wasn't the only "touched-out" tandem-nursing mother out there.

I found out I was going through PPMD through a friend I had met on Twitter and befriended on Facebook. She is a doula and midwife assistant, and the President of the International Cesarean Awareness Network (ICAN), Desirree Andrews. One day she was talking about PPMD, and the more I heard about it, the more I knew that was what I had gone through. I talked with her at length, and she played a huge part in my coming to terms with what had happened and beginning the process of forgiving myself.

Alyssa's Story

When I found out I was pregnant, and started reading up on all things pregnancy, I discovered the controversies around formula and breastfeeding. It hadn't ever occurred to me that there could be so many hurdles and debates surrounding breastfeeding, or breastfeeding in public! I started researching more and joined several breastfeeding support groups on Facebook including This Milk Matters (www.facebook.com/BreastMilkMatters), Unlatched (www.facebook.com/Unlatched), The Leaky Boob (www.facebook.com/TheLeakyBoob), and Breastfeeding Moms Unite (www.facebook.com/Breastfeeding-MomsUnite).

I had researched hospitals and obstetricians, and made sure to find not just a breastfeeding-supportive doctor, but also a certified Baby-Friendly hospital. I was not offered a single bottle of formula, I was allowed to breastfeed right after delivery, and was asked if I wanted to see an LC first thing in the morning. My son, Hayden, had a wonderful latch with almost no pain and was a great nurser, but when I looked at my son, I simply felt...nothing.

Thinking that it would pass, and the miracle of "love at first sight" that everyone else felt would eventually come to me, I continued to care for and nurse my son just as I should, but two days later, when I was released from the hospital, as I was trying to nurse my son back to sleep for what felt like the millionth time that night, I started to cry. Big, wracking sobs that I thought would wake my son's father in the next room. He had stepped up to take on the responsibilities of fatherhood, but would be stationed 2,500 miles away with no way to physically help out. I was going to be alone raising this baby that should be loved and cared for...but all I felt was anger and annoyance, and I could hardly stand to be around him. I felt guilt and a terrible fear that I would never come to love this child. Realizing that I must be suffering from postpartum depression, I panicked. I put Hayden back into his crib, grabbed my keys, and at 4 a.m. drove to the 24-hour supermarket and bought formula. I bought the first pack of ready-to-feed I saw, paid, and headed back to our apartment. When I crept back in, I woke Hayden's father and told him I just couldn't do it. I couldn't raise this child when I felt...nothing. I was terrified, not knowing what to do. I could hardly stand to be around him for all the guilt I felt. What kind of mother doesn't love her own child?!

We spent long hours talking and arranged to have his paternity leave extended an extra ten days. We contacted a lawyer that was a family friend, and decided that Hayden would return with his father to California. Signing over 100% custody of my child at four days old was one of the hardest, but best, decisions I have made in my life thus far.

Hayden received two bottles of formula, spitting almost all of it up, before I was able to emotionally handle the task of pumping for him. I may not know how to love the child that had grown in my womb for nine months and shared half of my DNA, but I couldn't let him suffer. I knew I at least wanted him to have breastmilk, and since my milk had come in, I needed to pump for physical relief anyway.

From then on, I pumped every two hours around the clock for the next ten days, and then I watched my son board a plane for California. I watched the boarding door close and tears once again streamed down my face as love finally overcame me. I dropped to my knees and quietly cried. My mother helped me up and held me as I tearfully promised to start psychological counseling immediately so I could regain custody of my child. I vowed to pump and send my milk, no matter the cost, so that my son could have the best that I could give him, even though that still didn't feel like enough.

For the next five months, I pumped milk and shipped it, paying about $150 for every 300 ounces I shipped. I struggled to keep up with his growth spurts. We had to resort to supplementing with formula the first three weeks he was in California as I reached out for advice and help from other moms online, and received both help and encouragement. Working with my son's father to have Hayden's bottle-feeding simulate breastfeeding, and with more help and support from mothers online, I was successfully able to have my son nurse without problems every time I was able to visit him.

My son is now six months old. I no longer suffer from PPD, and I have moved to California. Hayden's time is spent breastfeeding from me all day while his dad is at work, and having a bottle of pumped milk at night with his father while I am in class. Without the constant help and encouragement from online moms, I would have chucked away the pumping flanges and given up hope. Instead, my son is happy, healthy, and has no problems switching from breast to bottle and back again. Thankfully, he nurses like a dream, but I know he enjoys it most when it is right from the tap and we are cuddled in bed.

Chapter 12

The Unexpected While Pregnant

You can walk into any bookstore, head to the section titled "Pregnancy," and likely find multiple copies of *What to Expect When You Are Expecting* and other pregnancy books offering insight about the next 40 weeks of a pregnant woman's life. We expect pregnancy to be exciting and fun, and while there are some symptoms that mothers experience that are less than desirable, on the whole, it can be a pretty magical time for women. From the first time you see or hear the heartbeat, feeling those first little kicks and jabs, the pregnancy "glow," and grow the baby bump, it's a time when many women are fawned over, more than any other time in their lives.

What if this isn't your experience? What if you never expected to have the pregnancy you did? Is there a book that can prepare you for that? Of course there isn't. When the cute little maternity dresses hang unworn in the closet because you are too sick to leave the house, and baby showers wind up canceled because you are on bed rest in the hospital under the constant watch of a team of doctors and nurses—those are the events we never want to imagine will happen to us. We can't predict the paths our pregnancies will take, and for women who don't experience what is in the books and portrayed on television or the movies, these situations can be emotionally devastating. Beginning the journey of motherhood from a place of sadness or fear is less than ideal. I often tell women pregnancy and childbirth are like warming up for a big race, but the marathon really starts the moment your baby is placed in your arms. Making sure that we are as prepared as possible and in a healthy place mentally is really important, because motherhood is going to bring on a whole new set of challenges for which it is impossible to prepare.

Pregnancy turns many of us into information-seeking fiends, and the Internet can occupy untold hours of an expectant mother's life. Many women begin their online information gathering even before they are pregnant, while they are trying to conceive. So it only makes sense that they would stick around for the pregnancy and everything afterward. Thankfully, there are places women can go, resources that can guide them and help them come to terms with unexpected difficulties when pregnant, and most importantly, can connect them with others in the same position.

Tamara's Story

Somehow through a mix of my own upbringing and arbitrary standards forced on women to be "better" or "best," I went into motherhood with expectations that reality slowly crushed, sending me into a chasm of self-doubt. Then people—strangers—reached through the Internet and pulled me out.

My mother breastfed three children, used a food grinder to prepare fresh veggies, attended La Leche League meetings, and sat on the floor with me each afternoon fostering my love of language, reading, and singing. That's what I remember about my early childhood, and it was the standard to which I held myself. I never considered any other types of parenting because when I had my first son, I didn't know that "parenting" was now a noun, verb, label, and social microcosm just waiting to swallow me up. College wasn't that different from high school. Marriage wasn't that different than cohabitation. But motherhood and breastfeeding forever changed who I am, and how I view myself.

It took us seven months to get pregnant for the first time, and after two active, healthy trimesters I experienced preterm labor at 27 weeks. I was rushed to the prenatal intensive care unit and given fluids and medication to stop my contractions. My husband watched the monitor with a stoic face, almost willing the contractions to stop. I remember asking him how big a baby is at 27 weeks, and his answer was, "Not big enough."

That was the first time my heart swelled with the enormity that is motherhood. I think for most people, it happens the moment their baby is born. For me, that day was my introduction. It was heavy and scary, and I felt like my body was failing to do something that seemed effortless for other women. That prayerful day turned into ten weeks of strict bed rest and tocolysis. The days were long and fear-filled. With nothing but time on my hands, I paged through the bibles of natural birth and breastfeeding. I dog-eared pages on latch and positioning, practiced Kegel exercises, and tried not to focus on my weakening body and spirit.

Early in the morning just past 37 weeks gestation, my water broke. I leaked fluid from ruptured membranes for 12 hours without a single contraction, and as the intravenous Pitocin began to drip, my granola dreams for an un-medicated birth slipped away. I held on tight, almost to a fault, as induced back labor worked against my body, which was so weak after being confined to a hospital bed for the last 10 weeks. I got an epidural and delivered a healthy baby boy, who was placed on my chest smelling of tears and musky clay. Looking back on that

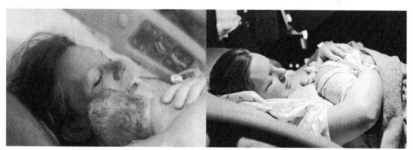

—photo credit: Sandra Reed   —photo credit: Michelle Hammons
Tamara meeting her baby boy after spending ten weeks on bedrest in the hospital.

moment, it was not joy that I felt; it was relief. His safe arrival was my biggest accomplishment to date.

Within minutes of his birth, I had nurses with blue gloves manipulating my breast into my son's tiny mouth. I felt clumsy and awkward as he refused to suckle. Over the next two days doctors, nurses, and lactation consultants bustled in and out of our room watching him cry, monitoring his climbing bilirubin, and commenting on his rapid weight loss. I remember one nurse rolled in a hospital-grade breast pump. She hooked me up to two small cups and told me to pump so that I could feed my baby colostrum. I turned up the pump and sat crying over those empty cups until I had abrasions on my areolae. I was given nipple shields, a supplemental nursing system, and breast shells. My feelings of failure culminated with my husband finger-feeding our hungry baby formula, doctor's orders. I had been a mother for less than 48 hours, and already I felt like I had failed him. People were examining me as if I was auditioning to be a mother: watching me struggle with nursing, with sleeping, with balance. I remember once we had our son home, I was trying to bring him to the breast before supplementing with pumped milk, and my mother said, "none of my babies ever cried like that."

Three days before my first Mother's Day, I got an email on behalf of my family outlining all of the ways in which I had failed my son. The letter urged me to put down the books and, "*… start relying on common sense and advice from the people you love. If breastfeeding is not satisfying his hunger then you need to give him a bottle of formula with vitamins and iron to help him grow. And believe me, breastmilk or formula, a baby will grow up the same way. You are supposed to be such an educated woman, start being a mother to this baby and take care of him properly …*" with a few jabs at the end about how my grandmother, of blessed memory, would be appalled at the mother I had become. You would have thought I was extinguishing cigarettes on my baby's arms while feeding him rat poison from my bloody nipples. That criticism burned like salt in my open wounds. I didn't need to be told that I was being a terrible mother when I was already telling myself that very thing every minute of every day.

I felt like both my pregnancy and birth expectations had slipped away, and I refused to give up on nursing. After a particularly frustrating day of trying to get my son to latch followed by finger feeding him milk and pumping every two hours, I posted a Facebook status about how hard it all was. A friend I hadn't talked to since high school messaged me with her story and offered me help and support. Then another message came in, this time from a college friend, again commiserating with how consuming it all is at first, but encouraging me nonetheless. People I hadn't talked to in years, even blog comments from people I had never even met—all cheering me on. These women were sharing their stories and encouraging me to nurse my baby.

I found a local La Leche League meeting, and was so embarrassed to attend with a baby who screamed at the breast. I sat through the meeting with my tiny infant in a room full of strangers telling their stories. I was amazed as they shared so many of the same feelings that had kept me so isolated. Meeting after meeting, I watched and shared, and learned not only to breastfeed, but to be a mother.

I found a weekly Twitter chat on Thursday nights called #bfcafe. Women used this hashtag all week to ask questions and share anecdotal stories and pictures of their breastfeeding journey. The women behind the hashtag–they lifted me up too.

My firstborn latched after 11 weeks and went on to nurse for 25 months, when he self-weaned. Those online messages, La Leche League meetings, Twitter chats, and blog posts got me through eight months of biting, chronic milk blisters, growth spurts, and multiple nursing strikes. At the same time, these strangers, friends, and strangers-turned-friends celebrated a love for nursing. They modeled parenting at the breast and helped me to revel in a motherly confidence that grew with each feeding.

Even after my son latched, I continued to pump, telling myself I would always have milk on hand for him should anything happen to our nursing relationship. He never drank a drop of my expressed milk, but seven other babies did. I pumped and donated over sixteen gallons of breast milk for friends and women I met through the informal milk-sharing community, Human Milk 4 Human Babies.

When my son was 14 months old, I became pregnant again. I lost that pregnancy at the end of my first trimester, but nursing helped me get through the foggy sadness. Every time I looked down, I was so incredibly thankful to have a healthy baby nursing in my arms. I knew after I miscarried that my milk would come back—I knew because I looked it up on the Internet.

I became pregnant for a third time this past fall. My firstborn weaned half way through my second trimester on his own terms. With this pregnancy, a lot of fear came flooding back surrounding my miscarriage, preterm labor, birth trauma, and nursing difficulties. I read through forums on the La Leche League website, reached out to friends who had a second child, and prepared myself and my body, for birth and breastfeeding. Research revealed I had birth options this time around. I learned how to work through my feelings of disappointment regarding my first birth and how to be optimistic about my second. I found a doula, talked to lactation consultants, and shared my fears online. I reached far and wide, and got back nothing but love and support in return.

I birthed my second son naturally in three hours and with only three pushes, in a hospital with the help of my husband and our doula. My body successfully carried a baby to 39 weeks, and I bravely and confidently gave birth to him on my own terms. They say you don't get a medal for birthing naturally, but you actually get more. I have never felt more powerful, confident, or feminine than I did on that day. I put him to my breast and he nursed without hesitation from his very first feeding. My firstborn made me a mother, and my second child made me an even stronger one. Each time I nurse, I am hit with an instant wave of motherly love and vulnerability that comes with seeing your children grow. In succeeding at this primitive task, I have gained not only two secure and healthy boys, but a mothering self-efficacy that can never be taken away.

Anyone who knows me knows that I am passionate about being a mother and about nursing my children. I have reached out to friends and strangers. I started sharing my journey through my writing. I shared my struggles, my triumphs, and my love for breastfeeding with the World Wide Web. I gave personal and intimate details of my postpartum anxiety, my birth stories, my miscarriage, and our weaning ceremony. I shared it all unapologetically, not because I am an expert on motherhood, but because I discovered that reading other women's stories is a vital piece to navigating the journey. I wanted to give back a small portion of what was given to me.

The upside to your own mother telling you that you are failing at motherhood is that nothing anyone says can ever hurt you again. I've supported, without judgment, women who nursed for six days and women who nursed for six years. I have shared my breastfeeding story over and over until that pain went away, and then I did everything in my power to help other mothers never have to feel the way that I did because I wasn't alone—and I never failed. I am so grateful to the women who reached out to me; Brooke, Megan, Lina, Ellen, Elita, Katy—and if I have helped one person nurse one baby during one moment of weakness, I've done enough.

We don't live in an age where upon giving birth, we can be swept underneath a red tent by our elders to learn by example how to nurse, love, and care for our children, but we do live in a time where honest, supportive, and knowledgeable women can be found at any moment of the day or night with just the click of a mouse. Just log onto Twitter while you are feeding an infant, bleary-eyed at 3 a.m.; someone else across the country is staring at her phone doing the exact same thing. The two of you are instantly connected. Reach out and share the journey.

Meg's Story

I'm a 31-year-old stay-at-home mother to three breastfed babies: a five year-old, a three year-old, and a 17 month-old toddler. I was an attorney, but while pregnant with my first child, made the decision to stay home. I am fairly open and comfortable with my body and with my role as a nursing mother, so I was never afraid or nervous about having frank conversations about breastfeeding, whether in person or online. I wasn't afraid to seek out help wherever I could find it.

My mother breastfed my two younger brothers and me. I don't know if it was normal for her contemporaries at the time, but I do know neither of my grandmothers breastfed. I don't specifically remember seeing breastfeeding as a child, but of course I did. I do remember that while my youngest brother was nursing, my middle brother and I would pretend to nurse our baby dolls.

While pregnant with my first, who was born in September 2007, I read every book I could get my hands on. I also did a lot of research on websites like *What to Expect When You Are Expecting*, and KellyMom. I always assumed I would breastfeed and honestly, perhaps naively, didn't consider any alternative. My husband and I went to a breastfeeding class run by a lactation consultant at the hospital where we planned to deliver Avery. The class was very informative, and I encourage anyone planning to breastfeed to take a similar class. The best bit of information that we took away from the class was that a woman needs a supportive partner in order to be successful. That certainly isn't always the case, but when things get tough and you are in pain, it is definitely helpful to have your partner supporting you and reminding you that you can do it. It is also helpful to have an extended network of friends and family who are also supportive. I was lucky enough to have an extended family that didn't bat an eye if I fed a baby in front of them. My brothers and father never made me feel uncomfortable or like I shouldn't be nursing in front of them.

I joined a "What to Expect When You Are Expecting" birth board. At first I tended to "lurk," but since then have formed lasting relationships with a lot of the women on that board. During pregnancy, I

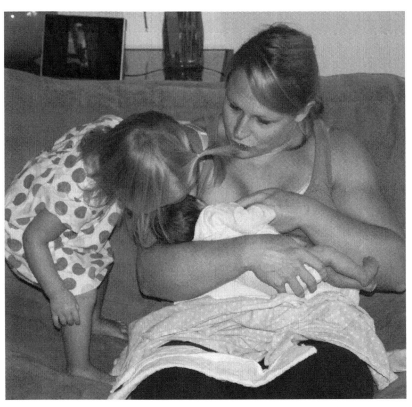

Meg teaching her oldest about breastfeeding, while nursing her second daughter. —*Photo credit: Meg Paulsen*

didn't feel ready to interact with them in a meaningful way, but read the discussions and tucked away bits of information for future use.

Due to medical reasons, Avery was delivered via cesarean section prior to my going into labor. She weighed 8lbs 8oz, and was beautiful. While I was being closed up, my husband went with her to be cleaned up in my hospital room. Immediately upon being reunited with Avery, the nurse put her on my left breast. A lactation consultant came in and deemed us to be on the right track, and after a few days we went home. Upon reflection, the latch was terrible and started a painful cycle that lasted a few weeks.

Once home, I was experiencing searing pain on my left breast whenever she would latch on. After some research, I decided to contact the lactation consultant who taught the hospital class. She came to the house, and spent an hour and a half helping me work on her latch; after a few days of hard work, things started to get better.

Those first few months of breastfeeding were difficult. Avery would not take a bottle and was a constant eater, so I felt trapped since I couldn't leave the house without her. Over time, I got used to having her with me all the time, and my parents, who live locally, would white-knuckle it while she cried on those rare times I couldn't take her with me. I always left her a bottle, but she refused to drink from it.

All this time, I would return to the "What To Expect ..." board if I had questions or needed some support. On the boards were women going through the same issues, or at least something similar, which made me feel less alone. Through some online research, I found a fitness group for mothers called Stroller Strides, and joined that when Avery was about eight weeks old. I also joined a playgroup I found through a hospital Web page and became friends with some local mothers, who are some of my closest friends to this day. There have been many emails and phone conversations about breastfeeding, both questions and advice. Having other mothers to support me in this journey has been essential to both my success and my sanity.

Avery breastfed until she was almost 15 months, when I weaned her. My husband and I had been trying unsuccessfully for a few months to get pregnant with our second, and I wondered if the breastfeeding could be contributing factor to us not having conceived yet. A few days before I ovulated, Avery didn't ask to nurse and I didn't offer. I became pregnant that cycle, two days after weaning, and planned to nurse our second baby who was due at the end of August 2009.

I went into preterm labor in July, and my obstetrician attempted to stop the labor using drugs. Unfortunately, that was unsuccessful and after 18 hours of labor, our second daughter, Paige, was born by cesarean section, weighing 6lbs 15oz. We gave birth at a different hospital, and their protocols were not quite the same. My husband went to the nursery where she was cleaned up while I was closed up. I would be reunited with Paige when I was moved to postpartum after being in recovery. We knew about this difference, and so my husband called my brothers so they would be waiting for me in recovery.

Once in the recovery room, it was discovered I was suffering from malignant hyperthermia, a condition in which body temperature quickly rises and severe muscle contractions occur; it was a reaction to the anesthesia used during the surgery. A code blue was called over the hospital address system. After pounds of ice and life-saving medications were administered, I was put to sleep so they could drop a central line in my neck. I was taken to the Cardiac Intensive Care Unit (CICU) so my condition and temperature could be constantly monitored.

The next morning, I was informed that the medications that were necessary to save my life prevented me from breastfeeding for 48 hours. I was devastated. I was really looking forward to those first cuddles with my newest baby girl, as I knew I should be the one providing her vital nutrients. I asked the staff to bring a breast pump to me so I could start pumping and dumping. The CICU wasn't used to having a postpartum nursing mother, so they didn't have a pump on hand. However, they found and brought me one. My husband convinced the NICU staff to bring Paige to visit me in the CICU, which was a brief and bittersweet reunion.

Later in the day, I was brought to the postpartum floor. Paige was jaundiced, so she was in a "bili box," which gave off an eerie blue glow. She was only allowed to come out of her blue box for feedings, which prevented me from really being able to cuddle with my newborn. I asked the nurses to bring Paige to me during feedings so my husband and I could give her a bottle. Some of the nurses tried to convince me to get some sleep and not to worry about keeping to a very structured pumping schedule, but I was too concerned about not building a supply for her when she could nurse, so I pumped when she got a bottle. The minute I was cleared to nurse, I latched Paige on. Due to her prematurity and her jaundice, she was a lazy eater. I was concerned she wasn't getting enough, and was advised to nurse and then bottle-feed expressed milk, which I did. A lactation consultant came to visit, but she basically said, "you know what you are doing, you have already successfully nursed a baby past one year," and that was that.

We had to leave the hospital without Paige as her jaundice levels began to creep back up, which was heartbreaking for us because we didn't anticipate having to leave her there. Luckily, the next morning she was released and she came home with us. Nursing was going okay, but she seemed very frustrated. She would pop off and cry out like she was mad, then she would start slamming her open mouth against my breast. I have a fast let-down and a very fast flow, so I was fairly certain it wasn't a supply issue. I consulted some breastfeeding websites, but didn't really find the right answer, so I contacted the LC who had come to my house after Avery was born. She immediately recommended a nipple shield, since Paige had been premature. She said that while Paige was big for a preemie, she was still a preemie, and probably didn't have the fat pads required to nurse well. I got a nipple shield and things started getting better, but she was almost orange at this point and I was still very worried about her jaundice.

I went to a local, LC-owned store that has a scale you can use to weigh your baby. I weighed her prior to nursing and she had gained the required amount of weight since her last weight check, which was a relief. Then I nursed her and re-weighed her, and all seemed good. Unfortunately, at Paige's next well check her pediatrician discovered her bilirubin levels were 25, and he admitted her to the NICU for light therapy. I cried while checking her in. She was required to be under the lights around the clock and was only to be taken out every three hours for feeding, which was against the on-demand style feeding I practiced. She had a couple nurses who were willing to bend the rules and would let her eat when she seemed hungry. I managed to pump enough milk for all her feedings, and if I wasn't there to nurse her during the daytime, the nurses would call and ask if I was close or coming in before giving her expressed milk. I felt very supported in my desire to nurse her during this experience.

After two nights, she was able to go home and we were able to leave the NICU behind us. She started nursing much better and gaining weight rapidly. In fact, she quickly became very chubby! Through some research, I learned how to attempt to nurse without the nipple shield to see if she was ready to nurse without it, and we were able to throw those away fairly quickly. She was less reticent about taking a bottle throughout her infancy, so I was able to leave her a little bit more than her sister, but for the most part she was my constant companion. When she was 17 months old, I discovered that I was pregnant with our third child, and she self-weaned soon afterwards.

My son Colin was born at 37 weeks by scheduled c-section on August 23, 2011, and everything went according to plan. The hospital, anesthesiologist, obstetrician, and I did not want a repeat of the malignant hypothermia episode, so this was a very controlled event prior to my going into labor. I had amniocentesis to make sure his lungs were developed and thankfully, they were, so we were able to meet our son soon afterwards.

Colin latched on well, and I kept him in bed with me almost all the time. He regained his birth weight by the third day, which the nurse said was pretty rare for a breastfed baby born by c-section. Of course, that made me feel good. While he developed a little bit of jaundice, we were able to do light therapy at home, and he no longer needed it after a few days.

I felt like an old pro this time around. There were no major obstacles like there had been with Paige, and I was not inexperienced like I had been with Avery. I felt confident and seasoned. I truly was able to enjoy him in a way that I don't think I did with the girls. Colin is now almost 17 months old, and still nurses a few times per day. I don't plan to nurse until he's two, but I also don't have a plan to wean.

A few generations ago, mothers did not have the wealth of information that is available online today; instead they had sisters, mothers, neighbors, or friends they could rely on. I feel like the Internet has become that community for today's mothers. Without social media like Facebook, blogs, websites like KellyMom, and forums, women might give up at the first obstacle. Instead, there is somewhere to turn in the middle of the night when it seems like you aren't going to make it until morning.

Tara's Story

My story is one of struggle, defeat, surrender, and finally of enormous change. Despite the challenge, I am forever grateful for the struggle because it shaped and changed me in so many important ways. I never intended to breastfeed. It was just something that we didn't do in our family. My grandmother was not breastfed. My mother was not breastfed, and I was not breastfed. We all turned out fine: smart and healthy. When my husband and I began to make plans to have our first child, breastfeeding was simply not part of the discussion. Why should it be? I was going to follow in the footsteps of the women before me, and formula-feed. Besides, there were more important things, I thought at the time: conceiving and pregnancy, and then of course having a healthy, smart, and "good" baby. I was determined to achieve those.

Preparing for a baby seemed pretty simple. My husband and I agreed that the time was right, so I began taking prenatal vitamins. I had my first experience with online support groups when I joined a fertility-tracking website. We were the September 2011 Baby Group, although at the time, none of us were pregnant. We were all just trying to conceive. During my "two week wait," I checked for online updates several times each day, and reported any and all potential symptoms that may indicate that I was pregnant to my fellow online group members. The wait was long, but the support of the other group members made it so much more bearable.

Then, one morning I woke up with a bout of nausea. I excitedly raced to the bathroom, where I received my positive pregnancy test result. I was three weeks and four days pregnant at the time. After sharing the news with my husband, I reported the news to my online support group. Congratulations were received, and I offered continued support to the other members who were still waiting for their positive pregnancy results. At the time, I remember being struck with how helpful my support group had become, especially during the dreaded two-week wait. It became very clear to me during this time that my real-life friends were not interested in every internal twinge, or any other possible indicator, that I might in fact be pregnant. However, my virtual friends were very interested in my symptoms, and I was interested in their symptoms. My online support group was offering each of us mutual reciprocity, and after all, that is the making of excellent support.

I was so impressed by my experience with my virtual support group that I decided to join an online birth club. My experience with my new group began in a very similar way as it did with my conception group. We were all in the early phases of pregnancy. So much of what was discussed involved sharing our excitement and fear of being pregnant, and reporting pregnancy-related symptoms. Not much else was discussed, and there was definitely no discussion of breastfeeding. If there had been, I would have assertively stated that I would be formula-feeding my baby. I had no idea what direction my life was about to take, and how the experiences over the next few months would forever change me.

A few weeks after I learned that I was pregnant, my symptoms seemed to be much worse than other members of my online birth club. My nausea, which I initially thought was cute, seemed to rage all day. I also began vomiting several times each day. At the time, I just thought that I had very bad morning sickness, and that it would eventually pass, and I did my best to tough it out.

One day, after vomiting everything I had ingested for the past several days, I fell to the ground and blacked out. I knew that something was terribly wrong. After being taken to my obstetrician for my first visit, I was told to go to the hospital immediately for fluids. My doctor diagnosed me with hyperemesis gravidarum (HG). I had no idea what hyperemesis gravidarum was, and honestly, I did not care.

All I wanted was to feel better, and I was sure that there had to be a pill to make me feel some semblance of normal again. My doctor and the hospital staff were kind and validating. I was given fluids and IV medication. After a few days, I definitely did not feel normal, but I did feel slightly better and was subsequently released from the hospital with a prescription for oral medication.

Still having no idea exactly what hyperemesis gravidarum was, and not 100 percent confident in the medication I was given, I returned home only to become extremely ill a few days later. I was re-admitted into the hospital, given fluids and IV medication again; that's when I realized there was no magic pill or any medication specifically designed to treat hyperemesis gravidarum. I remained in the hospital for a few more days and was released not feeling any better, but believing that I would be more comfortable at home. When I returned home, an overwhelming feeling of aloneness overcame me. No one truly understood how terribly sick I was feeling ... no one in my real life and no one in my virtual life. I was sad, depressed, and overcome by dark thoughts. I had no idea how would get through the next 30 weeks, and more devastatingly, I didn't know if I even wanted to.

That night, I searched online for any information on my illness and found an online support group for women suffering from hyperemesis gravidarum. I immediately signed up and began posting, asking for help, advice and, most importantly, support. To my amazement, I found an abundance of kind and caring women who were currently sick with hyperemesis gravidarum, and who were willing to support me. I was no longer alone. Even though this discovery would not make me better physically, the support did so much for my emotional well-being. My online experience did not end there. I reached out to another woman who had a due date close to mine, and we decided that we would become online support buddies. From that point forward, we communicated using an online source every single day. Her support and guidance saved me from a lonely and doom-filled pregnancy, and I am forever thankful.

One day during our online communication, she indicated to me that she was planning to breastfeed her baby. This was her second child, and she was regretful that she had not breastfed her first child.

She inquired about my plans: bottle-feeding or breastfeeding? I remember pondering this question for some time, and realized that something had changed; I had shifted. Maybe it was the 20lb weight loss. Maybe it was the fact that I had stopped taking my prenatal vitamins. Maybe it was the fact that despite not having to return to the hospital again, I had spent four weeks eating only ice chips, sipping sports drinks, and eating tiny pieces of pound cake. I knew that I was not ingesting anything of nutritional value and that I was malnourished. I also knew what this meant for my baby, and the risk that accompanied it. However, as I pondered that question I knew one thing: my baby and I were in the fight of our lives, and if we got through this fight, I needed to make up for the lost nutrition. I needed to provide for him, and the only way that I could provide for him was to breastfeed him. I knew that I would do everything possible to breastfeed my baby, so in my response to my online support buddy, I indicated that yes, I did plan to breastfeed my baby.

Due to the intensity of hyperemesis gravidarum, the focus of

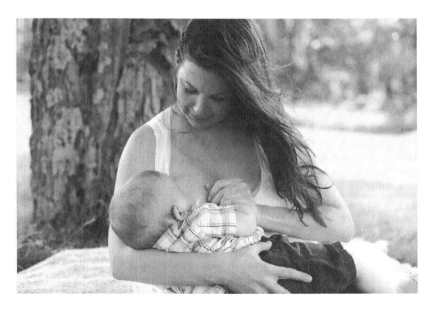

Tara breastfeeding her son, an act she never imagined would be part of her mothering experience until she suffered a debilitating condition while pregnant. —*Photo credit: Maxine Webber*

our pregnancy-related correspondence continued to be related to the immediate support of illness-related symptoms and emotions. Despite my affirmation, I didn't conduct much research on breast-feeding until after my son was born. Hyperemesis gravidarum is a debilitating illness, and much of my focus was on getting through the pregnancy. I remember thinking that I would figure everything out once my son was born.

Because of medical issues unrelated to hyperemesis gravidarum, I was scheduled for a c-section. A few days prior to my scheduled c-section, I woke up in severe pain. I remember experiencing the worst cramps I had ever felt in my life. I called my doctor and was told to come to the hospital. I notified my online support buddy, and she told me that I would be in her thoughts and prayers. I was in labor, and after about nine hours, my son was born. The hospital staff was extremely supportive of my desire to breastfeed, and after my son was born, my delivery nurse brought my son to me for skin-to-skin time. Shortly after that, my nurse brought my son to me and assisted us for his first feeding. He latched on perfectly.

For the remainder of my hospitalization, all of the nurses and a lactation consultant were helpful and supportive, and encouraged our new breastfeeding relationship. However, once I returned home, I realized I needed additional support. I was again alone in that, at the time, I didn't know anyone who had breastfed or who was currently breastfeeding. Because of my previous success with online support, I again turned to the Internet. This time I discovered my primary support through social media. These forums offered me the support and guidance that I needed as a new breastfeeding mother. I was able to ask general questions, as well as questions based on emergent situations. I always received feedback, usually within minutes of my posts. I was truly so impressed with how invested other women were in my breastfeeding success. I didn't quite understand the sisterhood at the time. I also spent a great deal of time reading articles and blogs of other women who breastfed. I was again amazed at the amount of knowledge gained and the level of support that I received during this time.

Through my daily perusal of the Internet for information on

breastfeeding, I began to learn more about Attachment Parenting (AP), and how what my husband and I were doing with our son seemed to mirror it exactly. It occurred to me that if I could find other mothers locally who also practiced Attachment Parenting, maybe I would finally meet other women who breastfed. In my search, I located two online forums on social media which, to this day, continue to be vital to me in so many ways—helping me breastfeed my son, parenting, and providing socialization opportunities for us as well.

These forums have not only provided me with support with breastfeeding, they have enabled me to have a social outlet with other like-minded mothers. There is such a high level of support for each other, and a collective sense of victory with each breastfeeding success story. These are women who donate milk to each other during times of need, offer classes and information on breastfeeding, offer childcare when situations arise, and do it all in a non-judgmental and compassionate way. I am honored and proud to be a member of these groups.

As for my story, I am happy to say that 16 months postpartum, I am still breastfeeding my son with no end date in sight. I continue to access my social media forums several times each day to provide and receive support, and most importantly, for friendship. I guess you could say that I no longer feel alone.

I believe that online support has been vital to not only the success of my pregnancy, but both my decision to breastfeed and my ability to breastfeed for as long as I currently have. The support and advice that I have received have been invaluable. In addition, as you may have guessed, my opinion on breastfeeding versus formula-feeding has completely shifted. With the knowledge I attained, I know how critical it is for a baby to receive breastmilk, and now I advocate breastfeeding for all new mothers. I have now become someone that people in my real world that are considering breastfeeding reach out to for knowledge and support. I am happy to provide the support, as well as my story of transformation. I believe that for me, I needed to experience all that I did in order to be led to the decision to breastfeed my son. Every day as I nurse my son and watch him being nourished by me, I am so thankful and grateful for the path that unfolded before us.

Chapter 13

How the Lactation Professional Connects: Why Social Media is Necessary for Today's IBCLCs

It's been almost two decades since women began to use the Internet to support one another, and there is obviously no turning back now. My hope for this book was to let mothers know they are not alone—to encourage, uplift, and educate. I also wanted to offer some practical information, not just for mothers, but for lactation professionals too. I discussed early on how women took the lead and embraced the Internet, making it work for them. It is important to note that this is where women are, and where they will continue to find information and support until the next major wave of technology comes through and surpasses the Internet in effectiveness. A technological overhaul of that magnitude may not happen in our lifetime, so it is important to hop on board this fast-moving train and get connected!

When I started my Web-based breastfeeding business almost three years ago, I knew that I needed to use social-media platforms to make professional connections. I am still amazed at how quickly it all happened and how those connections led me to a place where the connections became real-life ones, such as making face-to-face connections at conferences and shows. For this book, I called upon many of my professional colleagues for support and guidance, and for this chapter, I sought counsel from three IBCLCs who have really made social media work for them, and have used it to enhance their professional careers.

Lactation professionals first began connecting on LISTSERVs, such as LACTNET, BFAR, and Parent-L in the 1990s, as mentioned earlier. LACTNET still exists as a LISTSERV, but also has a Facebook group; BFAR has an entire website (bfar.org); and while Parent-L can still be found as a LISTSERV, its long-time members connect through a private Facebook groups now. Companies that market breastfeeding-related items know exactly where moms are connecting on the Internet, and are using them effectively to reach us. Lactation professionals are urged to use the same technology to support mothers, too.

> Professional organizations, including the United States Breastfeeding Committee, are calling on the International Board Certified Lactation Consultant (IBCLC) profession to bring evidence-based information to social media. In 2011, the International Lactation Consultant Association (ILCA) established a blog that received nearly 95,000 page views in its first year. Numerous individual IBCLCs, professional breastfeeding organizations, and mother-to-mother support organizations now provide information and support through networks, such as Facebook and Twitter (McCann & McCulloch, 2013).

If there was ever a time to embrace social media, the time is now, and it is easier than ever before to jump in the game!

Amber McCann's Story

Amber McCann, BA, IBCLC works for a community breastfeeding center and also does social media consulting and management. As a new mother, she found the Internet crucial to her very survival as she struggled to adjust to motherhood. Now she is able to employ it to reach mothers, but her perspective as a mother who felt saved by the Internet serves as a reminder of why the Internet plays such a vital role in growing and sustaining her profession:

> *I will always be passionate about meeting moms where they are,*

which, in this day and age, is online. As a new mother myself, I was very isolated from other mothers due to my physical location and, when I found a place online where other mothers were gathering, I felt like I had found a sanctuary. Even when I was unable to connect with my physical community, there was a virtual one (and I don't like the term "virtual"... they were very, very real to me) to hold me up and be my "village."

I suffered from very significant postpartum depression in my early months of motherhood, and there were many, many days when I was unable to get out of bed, unable to do anything except feed the baby. While I simply wasn't able to engage with my community, I did have my laptop, which could come into the bed with me. I would receive a private message or a message board post asking if I was doing okay. I would have someone just checking in with me. I'd never met these people "in real life," but very real relationships were built, and I am a better mother and a better woman for them.

My experience held professional meaning for me as well. When we embrace the "it takes a village" mentality, we, as breastfeeding professionals, should know that it also applies to us. There is incredible value in the collective knowledge that is the Internet. It affords us the opportunity to broadcast messages at a level that was previously impossible. It allows us to connect with other professionals that we otherwise wouldn't have had the opportunity to. It allows us to ask questions, get answers, debate, and brainstorm. Just as mothers shouldn't mother in a vacuum, we shouldn't practice as lactation consultants in a vacuum either.

With a background in sociology and a long-standing interest in generational differences, I've always approached my work with a mind towards what women of childbearing age are thinking, believing, and how they assign value and authority. We simply cannot have the mistaken belief that mothers think about things in the same way they did a generation ago. To do so doesn't give value to the incredible changes in thought and communication over the past years. On the flip side, to "throw the baby out with the bathwater," and not engage with and respect the incredible work of those who have come before us, is to miss the best resources we have.

Before my current position, I was in private practice. From the beginning it was incredibly important to me that my work was supportive of the life and family that I had, but that also functioned in a way that supported how new mothers thought about things and engaged with their worlds. The answer for me was to build a practice whose primary "storefront" was online, and particularly on social media. To be effective, my business had to be sustainable for me, and work with my life.

The one phrase that was the bedrock of my practice, was "What works for you is what works." This is true for families in the midst of breastfeeding challenges, and true for IBCLCs trying to figure out how to be relevant in the marketplace. We must take all of the information we have available to us and filter it through our experience, our knowledge, our abilities, and our limitations. I will share what worked for me. It might not be what works for anyone else but, for me, it was effective and allowed me to connect in a meaningful way with the mothers who needed my support.

One thing that is very normal for this generation of mothers is the blurring of lines between the "personal" and the "professional." It is a much different world in that regard, and I have found that often, they desire someone to "come along beside them" versus "walking in front of them and leading." They aren't looking for authority, they are looking for a relationship. I was willing to blur that line a bit, and share bits of myself on my page. I believe that doing so helped establish trust before a mother ever invited me into her home.

I'm a firm believer that not every professional is equipped to work with every mother, whether it be an issue of expertise or an issue of personality. By putting myself out there, my potential clients were able to decide if I was the right person to invite into their jumbled-up, postpartum world. Because they "felt like I already know you," we were able to work together in a more honest and vulnerable way. I didn't, of course, share highly personal details about my family and my life, but I did share the little things that might be connectors. I once had a mother tell me, "I chose you because you said you liked really terrible reality TV, and I knew you wouldn't think I was crazy to have The Real Housewives *on when you came." Score one for terrible reality TV! We shared a laugh and were able to quickly to get to the heart of her challenge.*

The platform I used most to engage mothers was Facebook, where I maintained an active page for my private practice business. I think it is absolutely critical that one decide what the "personality" of her business is. We often call this a "brand." I thought long and hard about how I wanted my business to be known, not just locally, but in a broader world as well. For me, my brand focused on empowerment, emotional support, and encouragement. I did this by providing evidence-based information, asking questions of those who engaged with my page, and sharing anecdotes and reflections from mothers who had "been there, done that." Other lactation professionals have Facebook pages with different "brands." There are those that focus on advocacy, those that share only stories from breastfeeding families, those that offer direct mother-to-mother support, and those that seek to be on the edge of controversy. Finding your voice in the marketplace is essential.

In addition to the general breastfeeding content I posted to my page, I shared practice updates, such as support group details, specials I was running, or local events. My page provided general information about how to connect with me, what services I offered, and how to find local resources if I was not available. It was the major hub of communication about my practice.

When I share about the use of social media in breastfeeding support, I am often asked about how to handle mothers posting their personal breastfeeding questions on the pages I manage. Based on my understanding of the ethics required by my profession, I do not answer direct clinical questions on social media. If a mother comes and shares her breastfeeding concerns on my page, I do one of two things (and maybe both!). First, I share relevant information to her situation, while being very careful to communicate it in a way that is directed to the general population. For a long time, breastfeeding volunteers and professionals have used the phrase "many mothers have found ..." to help generalize the information that they share. I also ask the mother to email me directly if her situation warrants further exploration or if she indicates that she's looking for more personalized support. From email, I can assess whether she requires specialized care or if I can help her find support in her own community if she isn't local to me. I also, with her permission, might share her question on my Facebook wall, which will allow input from other users of the page. With solid moderation, this is a wonderful source of support for breastfeeding families.

With social media, consistency is key. I try to post at least one item per day to my pages. By engaging with those who follow my pages, the content I share is more likely to show up in their News Feeds (the list of status updates that a user sees when they log on to Facebook). No one wants to see a constant "commercial" from an organization or business, so finding a balance between posts about services offered and information shared from other sources is very important.

If all of this feels overwhelming to you, don't despair. You are not alone. Fortunately, there are many IBCLCs already engaging with breastfeeding families online who are willing to offer their expertise, experience, and a helping hand. Don't hesitate to ask. We were once new to the medium ourselves at one point, and we want to help you along on the journey. Instead of pushing you off the diving board, we'll take you slowly into the kiddie pool. Mothers are having incredible conversations about breastfeeding online—would you like to be a part of them?

Robin Kaplan's Story

Robin Kaplan, M.Ed., IBCLC, practices in San Diego, CA, and in the last year has found a new way to use the Internet to support mothers with her breastfeeding podcast show appropriately titled, "The Boob Group." I used to live in San Diego, and long before I met Robin, I was aware of her fantastic reputation. When I had a dear friend who was struggling with breastfeeding and had exhausted my knowledge reserves, we called Robin to help get her on track with breastfeeding. Since then, Robin has grown her business and increased the level of support she is able to offer mothers by using social-media platforms. Like for so many of us, it was her own personal experiences as a mother that led her to the Internet, and helped her realize the value of online support:

My first experience with online support didn't begin with breastfeeding, although I wish there had been online breastfeeding support when I was nursing my boys over five years ago. Instead, I first sought online support when I found out that my son had sensory integration disorder (SID). For years, getting my son dressed had been a battle of epic proportions. The minute he put on a pair of pants or shoes, he would squirm and cry and throw himself on the floor, thrashing around. He was so uncomfortable, even in the softest cotton clothes I could find. Every day,

176

for about an hour, we would battle over what he was going to wear that day ... both of us ending up in tears and late for school. I knew that this wasn't "normal," but I also didn't know anyone who had ever seen this before. No one I knew, friends or family, had ever heard of sensory integration disorder and I was feeling completely alone, like I had nowhere to turn for support.

One morning, I had just had enough, and the stress was more than I could bear. I needed to feel like someone else understood what I was going through, and I truly needed some advice on how to deal with my son's challenging behaviors. I decided to look up Yahoo! groups for parents who had with kids with SID. That day I found three different Yahoo! groups and joined them immediately. Then, I just started writing. I posted a short version of my story, as well as a request for advice on where others found socks without seams (which were the bane of my son's existence). Within 30 minutes, I had multiple responses from caring, empathetic parents who offered words of encouragement, websites carrying seamless socks, helpful books and websites that explained what my son was going through, and HUGE virtual "hugs" for my entire family. For the first time in years, I felt like I didn't have to explain myself, and that I could easily access resources I so desperately needed.

So began my passion for online support networks. While having "in the flesh" friends will always be imperative for my personal well-being, most of my friends are in different stages in their lives. Each of us have things in common, but our kids are different ages, different genders, have different challenges, and we have different parenting styles and needs. This is why virtual friends and support groups are so critical. If I need parenting advice on how to deal with my seven-year-old with SID, I go to that virtual support group and post my question. When I need an alternative to antibiotics for an ear infection, I go to my "crunchy mamas" group.

As soon as I started my private lactation support practice, I knew I wanted to incorporate online/virtual support with my hands-on, in person consultations. I wanted to be available where mothers sought support and encouragement, and with two young children, it wasn't always feasible to provide support in person and over the phone. Texting and social media can be done "on the fly," and I can write for my blog after the kids go to bed.

For the past year, I have had the privilege of participating in the Breastfeeding San Diego group on Facebook, as well as serving as the administrator for the San Diego Breastfeeding Center and The Boob Group Facebook pages. Now, instead of seeking support, I am one of the mamas offering advice and experience, both from a personal AND professional perspective. I love watching the interaction between the moms in these groups as they share their experiences and knowledge about breastfeeding. They recommend websites and articles. They relate to and encourage one another. They help one another during this critical and emotional time as a new mother and it is absolutely beautiful.

Professionally, using the Internet and social media has truly propelled my private practice business to the next level. Clients can message me through Facebook and receive quick responses. Mothers I have never met in person can ask basic questions on my Facebook wall, or message me privately about a more detailed situation. Most of the time, I repeat a mother's question on my Facebook page so that other mothers can chime in with their recommendations, if appropriate. To protect myself and my clients' confidentiality, I had to create a policy that prevents me from committing a HIPAA violation, but that doesn't seem to affect my ability to provide online support. I am also very clear that I can only offer general advice (and I often add a link to one of my blog articles or to KellyMom.) Otherwise, they need to contact me personally and set up an appointment.

In addition to maintaining a presence through social-media platforms, I author a blog to which I regularly contribute. When I started my blog three years ago, it was to help my potential clients get to know a little bit more about me. I posted an article a month and it just kind of sat there. Then, I realized that day after day I was saying the same information over and over again to my clients. Rather than write this information in the client's plan of care, I found it was more useful to post it on my blog so that they could refer to it when needed. Plus, mothers from around the world could access this content, which made me feel like I was contributing to the greater good! Soon, I was writing about common concerns, breastfeeding toddlers, infant behavior, breastfeeding in the news, etc. I also started to include stories from breastfeeding mothers about issues like IGT and milk sharing. While there is never a shortage of content when it comes to breastfeeding, there are plenty of bad articles about breastfeeding on the Internet. My goal is to write articles that offer evidence-based recommendations in a non-judgmental way, for mothers to refer to in years to come.

To expand my reach in the Internet realm, in 2012, I helped launch a podcast called The Boob Group. Since we were creating it from the ground up, I had a few requests:

We had to be WHO Code compliant. No backhanded sabotaging of breastfeeding mothers would happen on my watch!

We had to provide judgment-free breastfeeding content. There is enough judgment out there to last a lifetime. My podcast had to be a safe space where mothers could listen to content, and feel supported and learn something that made their lives easier.

Social networking has provided me an amazing way to share my blog articles and podcast, and connect with other breastfeeding moms and advocates. The minute I write an article or upload a podcast episode, I share it through Facebook, Twitter, and Pinterest. What use is a whole library of helpful, breastfeeding-supportive information if no one knows it exists? Plus, I love when I see moms and breastfeeding-supportive businesses and pages sharing my articles and episodes when another breastfeeding mom is in need of advice, which is the whole point of creating this online content. It's creating conversations, connecting with one another, and providing a much-needed resource ... anytime, anywhere.

Fleur Bickford's Story

Fleur Bickford, RN, IBCLC is in private practice in Ottawa, Canada, and uses social media to disseminate evidence-based breastfeeding information so well that she travels to various conferences to speak about how other lactation professionals can do it effectively. On her blog, Nurtured Child, she shares her personal breastfeeding experiences and offers evidence-based breastfeeding advice. If you spend any time communing with lactation professionals through social media, either as a mother looking for support, or as a fellow professional, then you quickly learn she is very adept at engaging, supporting, and educating mothers through multiple platforms. Fleur shares wonderful insight about today's young mothers:

The stories highlighted in this book clearly show the profound impact that social media can have for parents who are struggling to adjust to life with a new baby, but what role can health care professionals play? Given that recent statistics tell us that 95% of millennials (adults aged 18 to 33) are online, with 80% to 89% of them using social-networking sites, it is clear that if we want to reach mothers where they are, we need to be on the social networking sites as well (Zickuhr, 2010, p.5). The Internet has become one of the first places that parents turn when they have questions about their own health or the health of their child(ren). Coming in just behind e-mail and search engine use, searching for health information is the third most popular online activity for all Internet users, ages 18 and older (Zickuhr, 2010, p.2). If we as healthcare professionals are not making use of the Internet, we are missing out on a huge opportunity to reach parents and have a positive impact on their health and well-being. Social media is unfamiliar territory to many healthcare professionals, and it can be intimidating to start with, but given its huge potential, it is well worth a try.

Many healthcare professionals wonder how it's possible to have any kind of impact with 140 characters on Twitter, or a short post on Facebook. One of the ways that we can make a difference is simply by pointing parents towards good, evidence-based information. The Internet contains an overwhelming amount of information and it's just as easy to find bad information as it is to find good information. The problem is that most new parents aren't able to immediately tell the difference. As healthcare providers, we are able to quickly distinguish between evidence-based information, and that which is based on opinion or questionable science. Parents these days are used to doing their own research and often all that they need is to be pointed in the direction of good information so they can educate themselves and make a decision about what is best for their family.

Social media is a powerful tool. Its reach is global, and due to its nature and the ability of messages to be amplified as they are shared, we are able to reach a far greater number of people than has previously been possible. Social media can be used to disseminate accurate health information and provide support for families; it is useful for marketing, professional networking and advocacy, but perhaps its greatest benefit is the ability to get feedback from parents. I have changed the way I practice as a healthcare professional based on the feedback I have received from my tweets, Facebook posts, and blog posts. Interaction with parents online provides wonderful insight into what their main concerns are, and how they perceive the information they are receiving from healthcare professionals.

If you are new to social media, the idea of jumping in can seem very overwhelming. There are numerous social-media sites, and they all function differently and have different strengths and weaknesses. The most popular social-media sites at the moment are Facebook, Twitter, and Pinterest. I suggest starting with one platform and getting comfortable with that first before trying to do more. Which one you choose is going to depend on what you would like to try to accomplish. Facebook pages are wonderful for establishing a community where you can foster mother-to-mother support and share information. Twitter works very well for networking with other professionals, and sharing short "sound bites" of information or links to more detailed information. Pinterest is a social-bookmarking site that can drive a lot of traffic to blogs/articles, and blogging is a great way to present more detailed information and receive feedback from readers.

There are a lot of options when it comes to social media. Some healthcare professionals are hesitant to interact directly with parents in such public forums. If this is the case, try using social media for professional networking to start with. Social media allows us to connect with healthcare professionals from around the world, and it is fascinating to be able to share and learn with a diverse group of professionals. If you don't feel ready to jump into actually using social media, there is still a lot to be gained simply by reading and paying attention to what parents and other professionals are talking about.

Social Media Tips and Tricks for the Lactation Professional

There are many online resources to help you get started with social media, but when reaching and engaging mothers effectively on topics as personal and important as motherhood and breastfeeding, one really has to be mindful of the tone of how the information is delivered. One of the best resources for getting started with social media is "Establishing an online and social media presence for your IBCLC practice," by Amber McCann, BA, IBCLC and Jeanette McCulloch, BA, IBCLC, published in the *Journal of Human Lactation*, October 2012. Highlighted is the need for IBCLCs to have a virtual presence, as well as tips for getting started with various platforms, such as Facebook, Twitter, Pinterest, and blogs.

Please check out the list below for additional tips and information, which is intended to be an introduction to the basics. Of course, you can always connect with someone willing to share their knowledge, try using social media to connect, or do more research online to find exactly what you need!

Basics of Facebook

Personal profile is your starting point
- This is where you can "friend" people, participate in groups etc.
- Good for interacting with people you know, or other professionals
- Pages can be created for interacting with moms/marketing
- When people "like" your page, your posts on your page (but not your personal profile) show up in their timeline
- Great for encouraging mother-to-mother interaction

Facebook Help Center:
http://www.facebook.com/help/

Facebook Guidebook from Mashable:
http://mashable.com/guidebook/facebook/

Basics of Twitter

- User's identified by @ symbol, followed by a chosen username
  o Examples: @NurturedChild, @TheBoobGroup, @VirtualBfing

VirtualBreastfeeding @VirtualBfing
Social Media can be a wonderful way to connect with and help
mothers who need #breastfeeding support!
Collapse   ← Reply   🗑 Delete   ★ Favorite   ••• More

An example of a tweet, using a breastfeeding hashtag. It's short,
simple, and effective!

- Users interact by "tweeting" short messages, sharing links,
  and "retweeting" (RT) messages from others
- Hashtags: put a # in front of any word to make it an easily
  searchable term, and allow you to reach people beyond your
  followers. Sometimes abbreviations are used, and most com-
  monly breastfeeding is shortened to 'bfing'
- Popular hashtags for breastfeeding mothers:
  ○ #breastfeeding, #bfing, #bfcafe, #bfchat
  ○ #parenting, #zombiemoms, #newmom
- Popular hashtags for lactation professionals
  ○ #LCchat, #ibclc, #LCinPP
  ○ #birthgenius, #doulaparty
- Lists can be created to allow you to monitor the tweets of
  certain groups of people. A great way to find people to follow.
- Applications, such as Tweetdeck or Hootsuite, make it easier
  to monitor hashtags

Twitter Help Center:
https://support.twitter.com/

Twitter Guidebook from Mashable:
http://mashable.com/guidebook/twitter/

Tips for Getting Started on Twitter

- Create a Profile.
  ○ Choose your username carefully and keep it professional.
  ○ Make sure that you fill in your profile details. Your profile
    is a person's first impression of you, so keep that in mind

and give it some thought.
- o Add a picture (avatar). It helps to give you an identity.
- o Remember that you are representing your profession.
- Keep personal details to a minimum.
- Consider adding a disclaimer.

Tips for Using any Social-Media Platform

- Remember that what you are posting is public unless you go to private message.
- Keep it professional. Re-read before you hit send.
- Keep religion, politics, and controversial topics, such as circumcision and vaccines out of your timeline, unless sharing facts.
- If you want to discuss controversial or personal topics, have a different account that is separate from your business one.
- Be prepared to back up what you share, include links to article or document, for example.
- Limit your use of short forms. Keep tweets/posts professional-looking.
- Be careful about what you share/retweet.
- Read articles before sharing.
- You are endorsing what you share/retweet unless otherwise stated (always check the page name, sometimes even ones that share interesting photos or links can include obscenities in the page name).
- Check that links are active/correct.
- Protect your space and moderate as necessary.

Cautions

- Information sharing only!
- Remember you don't have the whole picture.
- Go to direct message if you think the conversation needs to be private.
- Remind people of the limitations of social media as needed.
- Refer to healthcare providers.

- Healthy debate is great, but avoid negativity and arguments.
- Focus on the people who want to learn.
- If needed, agree to disagree or move to private message.
- Don't be afraid to unfollow or unfriend people that bring negativity to your timeline.
- Don't post that you are away from home/on your own.
- Don't feed the trolls!
- Beware of spam!
  - Spam exists on social-media sites.
  - Report as appropriate.
  - Use a spam filter on your blog.
  - Be careful what you click on. Don't click on links with no description.
  - Beware of private messages from people you don't know that contain links, or messages from people you do know that are not typical for them.

Important Things to Remember

- Keep it professional.
- Take the time to retweet/share other people's information.
- Manage your time.
- Balance marketing with information sharing/interaction.
- Have fun and engage with other people. Social media is about conversation!

Resources

Ask Dr. Sears: Dr. Bill Sears and his wife Martha have been helping parents raise healthy families for over 30 years. They have an extensive parenting library, have written countless articles for parenting magazines, and have appeared on television shows, such as *Oprah*, NBC's *Today Show*, and *20/20*. The site contains a great deal of breastfeeding-specific advice, and is updated regularly. www.askdrsears.com

The Best for Babes Foundation: The mission of Best for Babes is to change the cultural perception of breastfeeding, and Beat the Breastfeeding Booby Traps®–the cultural, institutional and legal barriers that prevent parents from making informed feeding decisions and that prevent moms from achieving their personal breastfeeding goals (whether that's two days, two months, or two years) without judgment, pressure, or guilt. www.bestforbabes.org

Breastfeeding Inc.: The World's Breastfeeding Resource, Jack Newman: Based in Toronto, Ontario in Canada, Dr. Newman runs one of the premier breastfeeding clinics in the world. His website and online videos are extremely helpful to mothers in need of assistance. www.breastfeedinginc.ca

Breastfeeding USA: Breastfeeding USA is a mother-to-mother support organization for today's breastfeeding woman. They exist to provide evidence-based breastfeeding information and support, and to promote breastfeeding as the biological and cultural norm through a network of accredited breastfeeding counselors, and comprehensive resources for the benefit of mothers and babies, families, and communities. www.breastfeedingusa.org

La Leche League International: Founded in 1956, LLLI has helped countless mothers breastfeed successfully. Their mission is to help mothers worldwide to breastfeed through mother-to-mother support, encouragement, information, and education, and to promote a better understanding of breastfeeding as an important element in the healthy development of the baby and mother. www.llli.org

BFAR: Breastfeeding After Breast and Nipple Surgeries: Created to support and educate women, their families, and healthcare providers about breastfeeding after breast and nipple surgery, this site includes articles on the surgical procedures involving the breasts, stories of women who have undergone these procedures, and forums to connect for more support than can be found through the information alone. Founded in 1998, and maintained by Diana West, IBCLC, and Carol Maranta, both of whom had breast-reduction surgeries themselves. Also has a sister site, www.lowmilksupply.org, to help mothers increase milk production. www.bfar.org

Breastfeeding.com: From The Bump and hailed as "the Web's largest breastfeeding content portal," this site hosts a wealth of breastfeeding information. Advisory a panel of experts includes Jack Newman, Nancy Mohrbacher, Catherine Watson Genna, and Jeanne Cygnus. With everything from breastfeeding basics, a community, videos, and more, it is a site used by nearly everyone, often a first stop on the web for a new mother looking for breastfeeding help. www.breastfeeding.com

Breastfeeding Basics: Anne Smith, IBCLC, is the mother of six children, and has been helping breastfeeding mothers for over 25 years. Her website answers many breastfeeding-related questions. Smith's site has been around for over a decade and is one of the most recommended for mothers searching for valuable breastfeeding support. www.breastfeedingbasics.com

Breastfeeding Made Simple: The companion site for one of the best-selling and most highly recommended breastfeeding books sold today by Nancy Morbacher, IBCLC, FILCA and Kathleen Kendall-Tackett, Ph.D., IBCLC, FAPA (listed in the recommended books section). The website contains additional resources, such as slideshows, videos, and handouts which cover just about every topic a breastfeeding woman can imagine. www.breastfeedingmadesimple.com

CafeMom: A website geared for the mainstream parent, with articles related to many aspects of parenthood. If you search for breastfeeding, you will find there close to 40 breastfeeding-related groups with specific interests from "Breastfeeding 24/7," "Breastfeeding Women of Color," and "Exclusively Pumping" mamas to name a few. www.cafemom.com

Dr. Jen 4 Kids: Dr. Jenny Thomas, MD, MPH, IBCLC, FAAP, FABM, provides evidence-based support to breastfeeding mothers. She recently co-authored her first book, *Dr. Jen's Guide to Breastfeeding*, and is active in promoting breastfeeding not only in her office by helping families, but in her local community. www.drjen4kids.com

InfantRisk Center: The call center at Texas Tech University's Health Sciences Center, specializing in dispensing evidence-based information to pregnant and breastfeeding women about medications: prescriptions, over-the-counter medications, herbs, vaccines, etc. IRC also advises on alcohol and substance abuse while pregnant and breastfeeding, nausea and vomiting while pregnant, and depression. Please call (806) 352-2519 for assistance and visit the website for additional information. www.infantrisk.com

Kathy Dettwyler, Ph.D.: As mentioned in the chapter on "Pioneers of Online Breastfeeding Support," Kathy's website was among the first to provide breastfeeding support, and contains links to her widely read articles and breastfeeding commentaries. If you need evidence or reassurance for yourself or those around you to support your breastfeeding choices, it is a wonderful resource as her work is thought-provoking and rooted in her area of expertise, cultural anthropology. www.kathydettwyler.org

KellyMom: This site provides support and evidence-based information on breastfeeding, sleep, and parenting. Founded in 1998, by Kelly Bonyata, IBCLC, this site has been a go-to for all things breastfeeding and it is usually one of the first recommended by mothers who know their way around the Internet. In addition to articles on her own site, KellyMom maintains a very active Facebook page, with a large following, as well as community groups that offer mother-to-mother support for pregnancy and breastfeeding support. www.Kellymom.com

LactMed: The U.S. National Library of Medicine offers an online resource (LactMed) for mothers to research medications and their compatibility with breastfeeding. There is also a free smart phone app that you can download to have the information at your fingertips. www.toxnet.nlm.nih.gov

Mothering: *Mothering* magazine was founded in 1976, and in 2011 published its last print magazine and became a Web-only company. The website reaches over 1.2 million mothers a month, and has hundreds of thousands of participants in its forums. Many loyal mothers are on-call to offer advice and support not only about breastfeeding, but about all things that tend to fall under the "natural living" umbrella. www.mothering.com

Postpartum Support International (PSI): Founded in 1987, this non-profit organization is dedicated to increasing awareness about the many changes that women experience in motherhood with respect to depression and anxiety. PSI has a far-reaching network of volunteers to support its mission. Find resources, newsletters, information on how to access help in your local area, and an emergency hotline by visiting their website. www.postpartum.net

The Leaky B@@b: A helpful blog with breastfeeding and parenting advice; The Leaky Boob has an active Facebook page with a fan base that offers constant mother-to-mother support. Founded by Jessica Martin-Weber, a breastfeeding mother, this site is a favorite of new moms and pregnant women looking for support. www.theleakyboob. com

Uppity Science Chick: Created and maintained by Kathleen Kendall-Tackett, Ph.D., IBCLC, FAPA, this is an entire website dedicated to a growing database of current and noteworthy research on the mind-body connection and how it relates to cardiovascular disease; diabetes; trauma and PTSD; depression in new mothers, and breastfeeding. www.uppitysciencechick.com

Women, Infants and Children (WIC): The Special Supplemental Nutrition Program for Women, Infants, and Children—better known as the WIC Program—serves to safeguard the health of low-income pregnant, postpartum, and breastfeeding women, infants, and children up to age five who are at nutritional risk by providing nutritious foods to supplement diets, information on healthy eating including breastfeeding promotion and support, and referrals to healthcare. www.fns.usda.gov/wic

WomensHealth.gov: A federally-funded website designed to keep women informed about breastfeeding, with fact sheets, breastfeeding videos, information about working and breastfeeding, breastfeeding laws, links to breastfeeding in the news, and postpartum depression and medications while breastfeeding. www.womenshealth.gov/breastfeeding

Work and Pump: For mothers who are working and need to pump to continue breastfeeding this is a fantastic resource. Founded by a working and pumping mother, it is laden with resources and tips from how to get started pumping, what to expect when you go back to work, how to prepare for pumping at work, and how to boost your supply. www.workandpump.com

Other helpful resources (birth, doula, mood disorders)

If you are pregnant and planning to breastfeed please take the time to think about your birth plans. Your birth story will be the first chapter in your breastfeeding book, so to speak. Consider finding a Baby-Friendly Hospital, which will support breastfeeding and not supplement your baby with formula unless medically indicated. You may also find that you want to have professional labor support (doula) or choose a midwife to attend your birth. As with breastfeeding, there is a plethora of support for pregnancy and birth online. Here is a list of resources to get you started on your birthing journey.

Pregnancy Information

www.pregnancy.about.com
www.childbirthconnection.org
www.evidencebasedbirth.com
www.VBACfacts.com

To Find a Doula

www.cappa.net
www.dona.org

Perinatal Mood Disorders:

www.marcesociety.com

www.jennyslight.org
www.postpartumstress.com
www.mededppd.org/mothers

Popular Breastfeeding Books

Gaskin, I.M. (2009). *Ina May's guide to breastfeeding*. New York: Bantam Books.

Huggins, K. (2010). *The nursing mother's companion, 6th edition*. Boston: Harvard Common Press.

Mohrbacher, N., & Kendall-Tackett, K. (2010). *Breastfeeding made simple: Seven natural laws for nursing mothers, 2nd Edition*. Oakland, CA: New Harbinger Publications, Inc.

Sears, M., & Sears, W. (2000). *The breastfeeding book: Everything you need to know about nursing your child from birth through weaning*. New York: Little, Brown and Company.

Spangler, A., Rivera C.A., & Powell, R. (2010). *Breastfeeding: A parent's guide*. Cincinnati, OH: Amy Spangler

West, D., & Marasco, L. (2009). *The breastfeeding mother's guide to making more milk*. New York: McGraw Hill.

Wiessinger, D., West, D., & Pitman, T. (2010). *The womanly art of breastfeeding, 8th Edition*. New York, Ballantine Books.

How can I find a Lactation Professional?

Lactation support is key to breastfeeding success, and we often need the help of other mothers with experience and an International Board Certified Lactation Consultant (IBCLC). Please visit these resources to help locate a professional in your local area.

International Lactation Consultant Association (ILCA): ILCA's website has a Find A Lactation Consultant (FALC) directory that is updated every two weeks and lists private practice as well as hospital-based IBCLCs. www.ilca.org

United States Lactation Consultant Association (USLCA): Like ILCA, this website has a FALC directory that lists private-practice IBCLCs, and it allows you to search by ZIP Code and distance from your location. www.uslca.org

Zipmilk: Currently only available for a handful of states, but the number is growing; to add your state, contact your state breastfeeding coalition to see about being included on the registry. www.zipmilk.org

Where can I find breastfeeding support groups in my local area?

Local support can be found through La Leche League, Breastfeeding USA, and your area breastfeeding coalitions. Inquire with your local hospitals and baby boutiques that carry breastfeeding supplies, as they often host regular support groups for mothers. For a complete list of Breastfeeding Coalitions in the United States visit the United States Breastfeeding Committee's website. www.usbreastfeeding.org

Are you interested in becoming a Lactation Professional?

Many women find that breastfeeding their own children gives them the desire to help other mothers do the same. There are many ways to support breastfeeding families. Here are some resources to help you figure out which area of lactation support might work best for you depending on your lifestyle, background, and interests.

International Board Lactation Consultant Examiners (IBLCE): IBLCE is the governing board for issuing the credential that requires the most training: International Board Certified Lactation Consultant (IBCLC). Obtaining this credential requires an examination, clinical hours, and coursework at the college level, as well as lactation-specific education. The website explains the requirements for obtaining the IBCLC credential and the various pathways you can go about it depending on your educational and professional background. www.iblce.org

For others looking to obtain a professional certification (CLC, CLE, CLEC) with fewer requirements and coursework, visit these websites that offer online training as well as options in a classroom setting:

www.breastfeeding-education.com
www.cappa.net
www.healthychildren.cc

Human Milk Donation

With increased awareness about the value of human milk for fragile babies, the demand for this precious commodity is increasing. As mentioned in Chapter 8, there are various outlets for donating milk. Donating is becoming easier as more milk banks and depots are opened, and more informal milk sharing resources are established. Please visit Human Milk 4 Human Babies and Eats on Feets to inquire about informal milk sharing (www.hm4hb.org and www. eatsonfeets.org). For information on locating the closest milk bank to you, please contact Human Milk Banking Association of North America (HMBANA), and see the list below for areas where you can help support mothers and babies with your donor milk. www.hmbana.org

ALBERTA
Calgary Mothers' Milk Bank
103-10333 Southport Rd. S.W.
Calgary, Alberta T2W 3X6
1 (403) 475-6455
Fax 1 (888) 334-4372
www.calgarymothersmilkbank.ca
contact@calgarymothersmilkbank.ca

BRITISH COLUMBIA
British Columbia Women's Milk Bank
C & W Lactation Services
1U 50- 4450 Oak Street
Vancouver, BC V6H 3N1
Phone (604) 875-2282
FAX 604-875-2871
www.bcwomens.ca
franccsjones@shaw.ca

CALIFORNIA
Mothers' Milk Bank
751 South Bascom Ave
San Jose, CA 95128
Phone (408) 998-4550
Toll Free: 877-375-6645
FAX (408) 297-9208
http://www.sanjosemilkbank.com/
mothersmilkbank@hhs.sccgov.org
mothersmilkbank@hhs.co.santa-clara.ca.us

COLORADO
Mothers' Milk Bank Presbyterian/St. Luke's Medical Center and Rocky Mountain Hospital for Children
1719 E 19th Ave
Denver, CO 80218
Phone (303) 869-1888
www.milkbankcolorado.org
Laraine.Lockhart-Borman@healthonecares.com

INDIANA
Indiana Mothers' Milk Bank, Inc.
4755 Kingsway Drive, Suite 120
Indianapolis, IN 46205
Phone (317) 536-1670
Toll-free 1 (877) 829-7470
FAX (317) 536-1676
www.immb.org
info@immb.org

IOWA
Mother's Milk Bank of Iowa
Department of Food and Nutrition Services
University of Iowa Hospitals and Clinics
University of Iowa at Liberty Square
119 2nd Street, Suite 400
Coralville, IA 52241
Phone: (319)384-9929
Toll free: (877)891-5347
FAX (319)384-9933
www.uihealthcare.com
jean-drulis@uiowa.edu

MICHIGAN
Bronson Mothers' Milk Bank
601 John Street
Suite N1300
Kalamazoo, MI 49007
Phone (269) 341-8849
FAX (269) 341-8918
www.bronsonhealth.com
Duffc@bronsonhg.org

MISSOURI
Heart of America Mothers' Milk Bank
At Saint Luke's Hospital
4401 Wornail Rd.
Kansas City, MO 64111
Phone: (816)932-4888
kcmilkbank@saint-lukes.org

NEW ENGLAND
Mothers' Milk Bank of New England
PO Box 60-0091
Newtonville, MA 02460
or
225 Nevada Street Room 201
Newtonville, MA 02460
Phone: 617-527-6263
Fax: 617-527-1005
www.milkbankne.org
info@milkbankne.org

NORTH CAROLINA
WakeMed Mothers' Milk Bank and Lactation Center
3000 New Bern Ave
Raleigh, NC 27610
Phone (919) 350-8599
FAX (919) 350-8923
www.wakemed.org
Suevans@wakemed.org

OHIO
Mothers' Milk Bank of Ohio
1132 Hunter Ave.
Columbus, OH 43201
Phone (614) 544-0814
FAX (614) 544-0812
www.ohoohealth.com
ffeehan@ohiohealth.com

TEXAS
Mothers' Milk Bank at Austin
2911 Medical Arts St. Suite 12
Austin, TX 78705
Phone (512) 494-0800
Toll-free 1 (877) 813-MILK (6455)
FAX (512) 494-0880
www.milkbank.org
info@milkbank.org

Mothers' Milk Bank of North Texas
600 West Magnolia Avenue
Ft. Worth, TX 76104
Phone (817) 810-0071
Toll-free 1 (877) 810-0071
FAX (817) 810-0087
www.texasmilkbank.org
info@TexasMilkBank.org

References

American Society of Plastic Surgeons. (2012). 2011 *Cosmetic plastic surgery and reconstructive surgery trends.* Retrieved from http://www.plasticsurgery.org/news-and-resources/2011-statistics-.html

Cassar-Uhl, D. (2009). Supporting mothers with mammary hypoplasia. *Leaven, 45*(2-3), 4-14.

Centers for Disease Control and Prevention. (2012). *Preterm birth.* Retrieved from http://www.cdc.gov/reproductivehealth/MaternalInfantHealth/PretermBirth.htm

Gray, J. (2013). Feeding on the web: Online social support in the breastfeeding context. *Communication Research Reports, 30*(1), 1-11.

Internal Revenue Service. (2011). Part IV – *Items of general interest : lactation expenses as medical expenses.* Retrieved from http://www.irs.gov/pub/irs-drop/a-11-14.pdf

McCann, A. D., & McCulloch, J. E. (2012). Establishing an online and social media presence for your IBCLC practice. *Journal of Human Lactation*, 28(4) 450–454.

Zickuhr, K. (2010). *Generations 2010.* Retrieved from http://www.pewinternet.org/~/media/Files/Reports/2010/PIP_Generations_and_Tech10.pdf